A Textbook of

HOMOEOPATHIC THERAPEUTICS

A Textbook of HOMOEOPATHIC THERAPEUTICS

With Clinical Approach

Dr K P Muzumdar

BSc, DMS, MBS, MFHom (Malaysia)

Visiting Professor, Shri Kamaxidevi Homoeopathic Medical College & Hospital, Shiroda, Goa
Emeritus Professor, Dr Babasaheb Ambedkar Marathawada University
Formerly Director, National Institute of Homoeopathy, GOI, Kolkata
Director, Central Research Institute of Homoeopathy, GOI, Kolkata
Chairman, Homeopathic Pharmacopoea Committee of India, GOI
Visiting Professor, Manitoba Institute of Homoeopathy, Winnipeg, Manitoba, Canada

New Central Book Agency (P) Ltd

LONDON

HYDERABAD ERNAKULAM BHUBANESWAR

DELHI KOLKATA PUNE GUWAHATI

NCBA

REGD OFFICE
8/1 Chintamoni Das Lane, Kolkata 700 009, India
email: ncbapvtltd@eth.net

OVERSEAS
NCBA (UK) Ltd, 149 Park Avenue North, Northampton, NN3 2HY, UK

EXPORT
NCBA Exports Pvt. Ltd, 212 Shahpur Jat, New Delhi 110 049
email: ncbaexp@ncbapvtltd.com

BRANCHES

212 Shahpur Jat
New Delhi 110 049
email: ncbadel@ncbapvtltd.com

Shop Nos. 3 & 4, Vinayak Towers
681/B Budhwar Peth, Appa Balwant Chowk
Pune 411 002
email: ncbapune@ncbapvtltd.com

Shop No. 15, Bharati Towers, Ground Floor
Forest Park, **Bhubaneswar** 751 001
email: ncbabub@ncbapvtltd.com

House No. 3-1-315, 1st Floor
Nimboliadda, Kachiguda, **Hyderabad** 500 027
email: ncbahydb@ncbapvtltd.com

GSS Shopping Complex, 1st Floor
Opposite College Post Office, Convent Road
Ernakulam 682 035
email: ncbaernk@ncbapvtltd.com

Radhamayee Complex (Second Floor)
Opp. SBI, Panbazar, Jaswanta Road
Guwahati 781 001
email: ncbaguwahati@ncbapvtltd.com

Textbook of Homoeopathic Therapeutics • K P Muzumdar

First Published: 2006
Reprinted: 2013

PUBLISHER AND TYPESETTER
New Central Book Agency (P) Ltd
8/1 Chintamoni Das Lane, Kolkata 700 009

PRINTER
New Central Book Agency (P) Ltd
Web-Offset Division, Dhulagarh, Sankrail, Howrah

COVER DESIGNER
Soumen Paul

ISBN: 978 81 7381 508 9

Price ₹ 135.00

This book is respectfully dedicated
to the memory of my late parents
Dr P. V. Muzumdar and *Mrs Ramabai P. Muzumdar*
who reared in me the qualities of compassion,
honest practice and service to the sick

This book is respectfully dedicated

to the memory of my late parents

Dr P.N. Mazumdar and Srimati [illegible] Mazumdar

who instilled in me the qualities of compassion,

[illegible] and service to the sick.

CONTENTS

CONTENTS

Foreword

I consider it a great privilege to contribute a foreword to this "Textbook of Homoeopathic Therapeutics" penned by Dr K. P. Muzumdar, a well-known stalwart in the field of Homoeopathic Education. It also gives me a sense of pride.

Advances in Homoeopathy has presented today's students and practitioners with a wealth of study matter and ever-increasing volumes in homeopathy literature. A busy student or practitioner may find it difficult to shift the desired necessary knowledge from this vast sea and may, therefore, lose sight of basic therapeutic approach to common clinical conditions which is of utmost importance in day-to-day practice.

Noting this insufficiency the author has put before the students and practitioners a concise and comprehensive text on Homoeopathic Therapeutics containing lucid therapeutic information to all common clinical conditions. The chapters in this book cover most of the aspects required for standard study of therapeutics and its use to practice in Homoeopathy.

I am sure this publication will prove quite useful to students as well as doctors. This is a book which is not likely to be quickly superseded.

Dr Arvind Kothe

Preface

The concept of this book has been made clear in the *Introduction.* The arrangement of the chapters are in the form of physiological systems and common clinical conditions mostly seen in clinical practice. Only those conditions which are amenable to homoeopathic medical treatment are considered here.Those requiring surgical treatment are not included. There are many other uncommon conditions which are amenable to homoeopathic treatment but not frequently seen in practice and, as such, have been excluded.

Conditions as seen in practice are described and nosological diagnosis is mentioned. Remedies which have a very close resemblance to the pathogenesis of the particular condition are described. It must be clearly understood that in Homoeopathy, the patient is treated and not the disease. However, there are many remedies which can be considered for a given condition but the final selection is on the basis of modalities etc. Rarely indicated remedies are not mentioned herein. Every homoeopath has his own experience and even if those remedies are not shown in the list that does not mean that they do not work.

The reader is expected to know the homoeopathic philosophy, the materia medica and the natural expression of disease in order to fully appreciate and reap the benefit of this treatise.

Acknowledgements

When I decided to write this book on Homoeopathic Therapeutics many of my colleagues and well-wishers offered to help me in collecting data, correcting my efforts and putting them into a shape. This was a maiden effort on my part to present a textbook in Homoeopathic Therapeutics to the students and practitioners of homoeopathy which are not available comprehensively in one textbook.

Notably I must mention Dr Mandar Patwardhan, BHMS, who was my assistant for some time, and is now a valued colleague. He was responsible for going through the manuscript and suggesting improvements wherever required. The other name is Dr (Mrs) Sneha Karandikar, BHMS, presently lecturer at Shri Kamaxidevi Homoeopathic Medical College and Hospital, Shiroda, Goa. I commend their efforts.

I appreciate the patronage given to me by Shri Subhash A. Shirodkar, Chairman, Governing Board of Shri Kamaxidevi Homoeopathic Medical College, for publishing this most sought after book in the field of Homoeopathic therapeutics and management.

I also recognise the efforts of Dr Arvind Kothe, Principal of Shri Kamaxidevi Homoeopathic Medical College for supervising the entire production of this publication.

I am greatly indebted to all of them.

Dr K. P. Muzumdar

Introduction

Institutional homoeopathy started in India more than 100 years ago. Syllabi drawn to teach in these institutions were also drawn roughly by then and there has been no significant change in that syllabi ever since. India is the only country where there is legislation for teaching homoeopathy at the undergraduate and postgraduate level. Practice of homoeopathy is legalized in India and enjoys equal status with other systems of medicine.

Homoeopathy was brought to India by Dr John Martin Hoenigberger in 1839 in the court of Raja Ranjeet Singh of Lahore. About 50 years later, in the 1890s, enterprising homoeopaths—followers of Kent and Kentian philosophy—popularised homoeopathy in to India—first in Bengal and then in South India. It is difficult to say who introduced the syllabus in the Indian colleges but the same has continued to be taught in the institutions even today, although many changes have taken place in the concepts of various subjects. Many attempts were made to change the existing pattern to suit the present day need in the field of medicine but it met with stiff opposition from a few with poor understanding and foresight and/or with ulterior motives.

Our approach to any disease involves knowlege of disease, miasms and susceptibility of patient. All these, when interlinked together, will give you more success in clinical practice. It implies in a true sense the Hahnemannian classification of diseases.

Our objective of emphasising on therapeutics is to improve the utility of Homoeopathic medicines in acute diseases or acute exacerbation of chronic diseases.

Similarly, although there is no change for about 200 years in Homoeopathy principles as practiced and advocated by Hahnemann (1755-1843 years) there have been considerable increase and improvement in the number of proved drugs, the techniques in its proving, knowledge in biochemistry and techniques in pharmaceutical science, as also understanding of human physiology and pathology. All these changes have made us to take fresh look at the therapeutic aspect of the science. The fixed principle of Homoeopathic practice still remains '*Let Likes be treated by Likes*'. With this in view the concept revolves round the patient. The treatment, therefore, is also oriented round the patient rather than round the disease—unlike in conventional medicine. In other words, Homoeopathy treats the patient and not the disease.

No doubt we value our old literature, our elders and their wisdom. Yet we have to change our philosophical thinking to accommodate the newer additions or changed thinking. What we are taught and what we read presently in terms of homoeopathic therapeutics needs a second look. Therapeutics is described in all the standard books of today, a list of drugs and their symptoms alphabetically arranged under a disease condition. That does not give adequate understanding to the reader. In fact, the therapeutics should be based on the different phases of the disease expressed by the patient—as they appear during the course of that condition.

I have, therefore, tried to modify the concept of treatment on those lines. A case is received by the physician with all its signs and symptoms—they assist a reader to recall remedies in the materia medica, mental assessment of the patient in terms of its miasmatic status, and correlation of the signs gathered on examination of the patient —in fact what exactly one would be doing in practice or at the bedside. It is only then one would try to fix the phase of the disease, select the remedy on getting this additional information of signs and symptoms and data from his questioning and examination of the patient. The doctor can analyse and synthesise the case to prepare his all-comprehensive picture of totality the most suitable and find an appropriate remedy. The diagnosis or the name of the disease of the presenting complaint has been given to assess the prognosis and diet.

Homoeopathic Therapeutics is a vast and complicated subject—each case needs to be considered from different angles. Although totality is the ideal, a case can be studied from different approaches—causation, characteristic modalities, miasmatic consideration and uncommon signs and symptoms. The remedies mentioned for various conditions in the text are gross which have similar pathogenesis to the disease conditions. Sound knowledge of natural history of medicine, materia medica, and the repertory is therefore essential.

In this treatise I have considered those conditions which are frequently met with in practice and which are amenable to Homoeopathic medical treatment. But there are few conditions which look like incurable often do resolve with success. There are many uncommon conditions those have been left out or those needing surgical interventions have not been considered. One should remember that there have been cases requiring surgical intervention have been resolved through homoeopathic treatment without the use of a knife. Similarly many uncommon conditions have been treated by homoeopathy otherwise thought to be incurable which have shown miraculous cures in the hands of an artistic homoeopath.

Dr K.P.Muzumder

1 PYREXIA

- Definition
  Types of Pyrexia
- Symptomatology of Pyrexia
- Investigations, Treatment and Management
- Presentation of cases with fever, Causes of Ppyrexia
- Diet

In healthy person body temperature is regulated between 35.8° to 37.2°C. (96.5 to 99°F). There is a diurnal variation to the temperature. The temperature is at lower level in the morning and increases as the day rises. This variation is seen in fevers also.

Pyrexia is a condition of raised body temperature (taken in mouth) which is above 37.7° C. The condition is normally called 'febrile'.

Types of pyrexia : In the absence of eruption, the only guide to pyrexia is the course of temperature. There are three types of pyrexia based on the course of temperature that pursues on day-to-day basis:

(i) *Continued fever :* The temperature remains elevated for most of the time and the variation does not exceed more than 1° to 1.5°.

(ii) *Remittent fever :* Here the variation is more than the diurnal and it does not touch the normal.

(iii) *Intermittent fever :* Here the temperature at some time of the day is normal and at other time of the day is higher, it is raised by one, two or more degrees.

(iv) *Compound fever :* Boenninghausen has coined a fourth type of fever called 'Compound Fever', unlike the other fevers where the stages are chill→ fever → sweat that follow each other. Boenninghausen has observed that there is class of fevers in certain individuals where this regularity of chill, heat and sweat is not maintained. But instead the fevers begin with chill, shivering or with sweat, or with dry heat fever.

Causes of pyrexia

There are two main causes of Fever : (i) Infectious. (ii) Non-infectious

Fever in infection may be due to either a bacterial or endogenous pyrogen liberated from the polymorphs or other tissues as a result of bacterial action. Fever may be absent if the inflammation is localized as in case of small boil or any dormant and inactive chronic infection such as tuberculosis.

Fever is often present in neoplastic diseases, in hypersensitive reactions including those induced by drugs, and immunological disorders — especially those involving connective tissues; renal or pancreatic carcinoma, primary or metastatic carcinomata of the liver or lungs are liable to induce high fever, polyarteritis, systemic lupus erythematosis, acute rheumatic fever, rheumatoid arthritis and progressive systemic sclerosis are examples of immunological disorders where there is variable degree of fever.

Fever frequently follows injuries, severe haemorrhages, venous or arterial thrombosis, embolism and infarction of tissues. Fever may accompany severe anaemia where the Hb is less than 4g/100ml and hyperthyroidism. Fictitious fever is one that is created by patient or his attendants by cleverly manipulating the thermometer readings through hot water bottles etc.

In homoeopathic parlance the cause of the fever paroxysm is due to the transitory outburst of latent psora. As a rule, family history is more important than the actual signs present with the fever. Determination of constitutional miasm is very important since the severity of relapsing tendencies of that attack of paroxysm depends on these miasmatic background. The experience of the elders show that if the remedy is selected on the basis of the totality of subjective, objective, and miasmatic symptoms the patient may be cured in any stage of the fever. It is not necessary for the fever to run its course. Another cause of the intermittent fever is found in the inherited dyscrasia of the patient — psoric and tubercular diathesis. All the fevers then tend to a protracted, low or malignant type, which occur in the psoric or tubercular patient, and more deeply psoric it is, more malignant is the attack.

Symptomatology of pyrexia

In some instances the pyrexia may be attended with no symptoms but in almost all cases where the temperature is being elevated the patients complain of feeling of "chill" or shivering or rigors. At times there is burning hot feeling. Headache, restlessness and vague pains in the limbs and back are also common.

Weakness and malaise is present. Skin is hot and dry to touch, with rapid pulse and respiration.

Skin rash is often present with macular, papular, vesicular and pustular eruptions. The rashes are very distinctive of different diseases like measles, chicken pox or scarletina etc.

Appetite is poor, tongue furred and bowels are constipated. Urine is highly coloured and scanty.

In children, vomiting and convulsions may herald an attack of pyrexia.

Following useful facts may be remembered regarding temperatures :

(i) A sudden advent of high temperature in a previously healthy person without other pointing symptoms indicates Influenza, Tonsillitis, Scarlet fever, Pneumonia or Urinary infection.

(ii) A very gradual advent of fever is suggestive of Tuberculosis, and, sometimes Typhoid fever.

(iii) A fresh rise of temperature after it has begun to fall indicates a complication or relapse.

(iv) A sudden fall in temperature during the course of fever may indicate haemorrhage, perforation, or profuse diarrhoea.

(v) In non-febrile conditions like tetanus, delirium tremens, cancer, epilepsy, apoplexy, cholera etc., if there is a rise of temperature it generally indicates a fatal termination.

Investigations

Although investigations may not help us in selection of the remedy, the procedure is essential in order to determine the cause of fever, the prognosis of the case, and advice of diet.

It is observed today that physician orders all types of tests, whether they are essential or not. Only appropriate tests should be ordered. Where the diagnosis is obvious no tests may be necessary.

Complete Blood Count (CBC) :This often gives a guide to the type of infection. Polymorphonuclear leucocytosis indicate bacterial infection.

Neutropenia: Indicates viral infection, brucellosis, typhoid, overwhelming septicaemia.

Lymphocytosis: Viral infection, whooping cough. Atypical lymphocytes: Infectious mononucleosis. Eosinophilia: Parasitic infections, helminthiasis, allergic state.

ESR and C-reactive proteins: are raised

Liver biochemistry: is often slightly abnormal in infections. Serum transferases are also raised in hepatitis and other liver infections.

Urine Analysis: should be done even if there is no indication or absence of symptoms and signs.

Chest X-Ray: Often it may reveal a small patch of pneumonia, pleurisy, or a neoplastic growth.

Specialized investigations can be carried out only to make specific diagnosis such as blood culture, CSF, imaging procedures like CT Scan, sonography etc.

Treatment and Management

Fever is one of the most common conditions we come across in our daily practice. Our approach to fevers — from therapeutic point of view — is different from the one held by conventional medicine. The entire therapeutic exercise depends upon the onset, the pace and direction of its progress, associated complaints like chill, heat, and sweat stage and, above all, the constitution of the individual presenting the condition.

Fever is, a result of sudden outburst of the latent Psoric state. Some fevers start suddenly but others start slowly and develop into full blown much later. The sudden development of fever belongs to Psoric and Tubercular constitution whereas the slow developing picture belongs to Sycotic constitution. Tendency to relapse is found in all acute diseases and in most fevers. This outburst of latent psora assumes a periodicity occurring every 3-5-7-14- 21-28 days and pertains to the patient and not to the fever. In the mild forms, it is this periodic return of the paroxysm to which the name quotidian, quartan, tertian etc. has been given. In typhoid, typhus fevers, and some malarial fevers the relapse assumes a weekly or monthly aggravation.

The first prescription on totality of the symptoms of any febrile attack may be Aconite, Arnica, Baptisia, Belladonna and so on, it may not only remove the group of symptoms for which it was given but apparently restore, the health of the patient when the original cause still remains uncured and produces a return of fever. After the first relapse, when the symptoms are taken for second prescription, the lines of comparison must be extended so as to include the *miasm* — the inherited tendency — and the family history should be carefully examined for here we will find the key to unlock the tendency. In practice, we experience "complaints that are continuously relapsing." Sulphur is often indicated and prescribed. When Sulphur or the best selected remedy fails to relieve or permanently improve, Psorinum or Tuberculinum — selected upon the symptoms and the peculiarities of the family history and inherited diathesis — will cut short the acute attacks and prevent a future relapse.

If we examine the literature and critically go through the writings of the elders we see the wisdom in their observations. They have grouped the drugs according to their expressions seen in the first, second, and third week of fever :

1. Patient complains of sudden development of chill followed by acute, sudden and violent invasion with fever. This is caused by exposure to dry cold winds, draft of cold air, or checked perspiration, at times during hot weather. Thirst and restlessness with anxiety, fear, and exalted sensibility are its leading indications Drenching sweats often relieves all complaints. **Aconite nap** is indicated.

2. Patient comes down with sudden congestion, furious excitement, and perverted special senses. The skin is hot, red and flushed, throbbing carotids, pupils are dilated with blood-shot eyes. In spite of all this there is comparative absence of toxaemia. Indicates **Belladonna.** Clinically, it is found useful in scarlet fever in lower potency — both as curative and prophylactic: with red throat, hot and dry, nausea and vomiting, with hot head or delirium.

3. Patient complains of developing fever during dentition, or after getting wet while perspiring, restlessness with continuing change of position, finds difficult to remain in bed usually at night, associated with severe muscular pains with constant desire to stretch. There is alternate chill and heat with flushing of skin, shining texture. Indicates ***Rhus toxicodendron***. Clinically found useful in erysipelas and vesicular rash

with the beginning of fever, simulating rash of Chicken pox. It also has measly and urticarial rash on the body with the fever which passes off with the development of sweat.

4. Patient usually complains of paroxysms of fever in the morning. There is thirst several hours before the chill develops and it continues during the chill and during the heat stage too. And although there is heat there is no sweat. Vomiting is present with the drinking. In fact, this symptom is more important than the bone pains. Indicates ***Eupatorium perfoliatum.***

5 Muscular soreness, great soreness, prostration and headache. Anticipatory anxiety due to unusual ordeal, bad news, grief, or fear hastens the chill. This is followed by heat around the face and head and chill along the spine. He complains of staggering and incoordination of muscles. There is imperceptible and slow pulse. This gives an indication of ***Gelsemium***. He also recalls that there was a similar attack the previous winter and also at times in-between without chill. Peculiarity of this is there is no thirst during the heat stage but has thirst during the sweat stage. There are more of remittent fevers than intermittent. In addition, the patient has profuse urination. The apyrexial stage of these patients is of prostration. This is indicated in septic and intermittent fevers. It is extremely useful in Measles with typical catarrhal symptoms, involving eyes, nose and throat, with great prostration. Early stage of typhoid with vertigo and great weakness and chilliness in the back, low type of scarlet fever and mild form of erysipelas.

6. Patient had cold and overripe fruits, icecream, sour beer, bad sausages or strong cheese — in short had created a derangement in the stomach that brought on the fever. Although there is fever and burning within, the body is externally cold. There is frequent thirst, fear, restlessness. There is typical shivering in the morning with heat by 2 p.m. There is marked periodicity — either daily or every alternate day. These symptoms highlight **Arsenic alb.** The chill and chilliness is without thirst but occasionally there is thirst for hot water. This is indicated in Malarial fevers with great prostration. Great variety of intermittent fevers with inequality between three stages. In low type of typhoid fever with Arsenic characteristics. In Typhus fever, blood poisoning, with tendency to disorganization of blood and other tissues. In haemorrhagic measles, eruptive fevers and in scarlet fever.

7. Patient complains of fever developing after drinking iced water or eating cold food, particularly after getting heated in the sun or warm and sultry atmosphere or exposure to draft of cold wind. Patient may even complain of development of fever after chagrin, mortification, or anger. The fever accompanies headache, bodyache, stitching pains and aggravated by slightest movements. All these point to **Bryonia**. It is indicated often with all the characteristic symptoms in febrile state, in scarlet fever or measles or any inflammatory condition of any organ and tissue if headaches, thirst and aggravation by motion is present.

8. Patient reports with a peculiar chill and shivering in the morning, generalized weakness in the limbs, aggravated by walking in the open air, heat stage alternated in the afternoon. All the three stages are well-marked. Preceding the chill has violent

thirst and violent headache. The sweat is profuse, causing debility. He complains that once the fever recedes there is great weakness with ringing in the ears and emptiness in the stomach This is the intermittent fever of **China.**

9. There is a complaint that the chill often begins at 10-11a.m.,with thirst and pain; drinking does not relieve the thirst but profuse sweat relieves all the symptoms. Throbbing headache often accompanies the chill and fever .At times there are loose stools (Malaria). The onset of fever will produce intense itching on the body. **Natrum mur** has typical intermittent fever with headache.

10. Patient has slow and low grade temperature with weary and bruised feeling all over the body. Pain and tenderness in the right iliac area and generalized soreness of the abdomen. There is dusky face, offensive breath, slow pulse and restlessness; development of chill in the back mostly in the evening; sensation of suffocation and wants to loosen his clothes at the neck, heat is as if from the orgasm. **Lachesis** has periodicity, mostly developing in spring.

11. Fever is usually due to respiratory infection like pneumonia, or bronchitis that may convert into tubercular infection. The chill is alternating with heat, and shivering in the evening without thirst. There is sweat all over the body in the morning. Patient is extremely sensitive to noise.

12. Fever brings on great debility, stupor and diarrhoea, rattling mucus in the chest, this mostly in Typhoid fever. There is quite delirium, disconnected talk, extremities are cold and discharges are involuntary. Although the temperature is low there is nose bleed, and involuntary, undigested stool, milky and albuminous urine in **Phosphoric acid.**

13. Patient has a profound prostration, mouth full of ulcers, intermittent pulse and involuntary stools. Typhoid fever of very low stupid type, involuntary discharges and prone to bed-sore. Often there is low type of remittent fever. Indicates **Muriatic acid.**

14. Fever that follows after septicaemia, puerperal or post-surgical manipulations. Severe bone pains in limbs. Heat is so sudden rising with temperature that the pulse is out of proportion to fever, and abnormally rapid. This powerful nosode overrides other similar drugs. It is indication of **Pyrogen.**

15. Generally catarrhal fever or any other gastric or bilious fever, patient being sensitive to cold, tongue is flabby and clean or light-coated offensive. Has a nocturnal aggravation. Hectic fever, creeping chill and perspiration does not relieve the temperature, although there is tendency to free perspiration. It is **Mercurius.**

It is essential to determine the **Fever totality** to arrive at a right remedy.

The cause, — ailment from, — the Chill and its various time modalities, any characteristic sign or symptom and its concomitant; and, most important, the apyrexial picture. All these will constitute Fever Totality.

In **Psoric** disposition the response would be very quick, even the development of true fever picture will be sudden and fast. Whereas, in **Sycotic** disposition, the responses will be slow in establishing the fever in its true sense. Even the speed with which the remedy acts will be slow and tardy. In **Psoric** and **Tubercular** dispositions there will be marked periodicity as in cases of intermittent fevers. In Syphilitic fevers there will be destructive pathology and disturbed immune mechanism including malignancy.

Routinely three points must be investigated in a case of pyrexia :

(1) Leading symptoms complained by the patient. (2) History of the illness. Precise duration of the illness is very important. Majority of fevers usher suddenly and with rigors and chills but few of the fevers like typhoid and diphtheria commence insidiously. The day of the fever must always be borne in mind so that one is aware of what to expect next. (3) The examination of the patient in general — any development of rash? The temperature and its course.

Every organ must be systematically and carefully examined as the patient's condition may permit in order to either detect or to exclude any local disease. This is important because all cases of fevers are associated with or due to some local inflammatory disease or some generalized febrile disorder, e.g. typhoid fever.

Presentation of cases with fever

1. ***A person comes down suddenly with fever after exposure to dry cold winds or getting the perspiration checked, and with dry hot skin, restlessness and anxiety.***

Sudden burning fever developing after dry cold wind exposure, unquenchable thirst, mental restlessness and anxiety will point to **Aconite.**

Sudden high fever, hot head, icy cold feet, often ending in the delirious state. The heat is burning, steaming, there is no thirst with fever. There is fullness and congestion with throbbing pains. The pupils are wide dilated. Useful in Scarlet fever, red throat, hot and dry skin, nausea and vomiting. Rarely useful in typhoid fever, Often useful in dentition fever, and any form of malarial fever will indicate **Belladonna.**

Sudden development of chill, in the day-time, and thirst, in the evening, heat on the face, shivering in the morning alternating with heat — there is periodicity of these attacks. Very deep acting remedy affecting every organ and tissue. There is all-prevailing anxiety, exhaustion, and restlessness. High and hectic fever, but the body cold as ice, cold sweats, coldness is in spots. Although sensitive to cold yet better in open air. There is aggravation during midday and midnight. Prophylactic for yellow fever. Transforms into intermittent fever. Thirst for little quantity of water at intervals. There is great periodicity daily, every alternate day, every two days, every week, every fortnight, or every year. This points to **Arsenic alb.** Arsenic alb. works as a prophylactic for Yellow fever and also transforms into Intermittent fever.

2. ***Patient gets fever with bodyache after getting heated in the sun and then getting wet in the rain while still perspiring.***

This indicates **Bryonia alba:** the fever is accompanying typical headache, thirst and the intolerance of motions. The body is dry hot. This febrile state often accompanies some inflammatory process in various organs and tissues. Also we find the indication of Bryonia with sudden chilliness after a midday nap, with confusion in the head, or while walking with heat, mostly towards the evening, thirst, and hot and red cheeks. Frequently indicated in scarlet fever, or when the eruption of the eruptive fevers do not develop.in time. In typhoid fever it is often indicated, in the early stages with occipital headache, furred tongue, thirst, and abdominal soreness, typhoid marked with gastro-hepatic complications.

Ailment from getting wet while still perspiring — there is creeping chilliness, on waking and rising in the morning and in the afternoon with heat and malaise, bodyaches which aggravates on first movement but comparatively better once he starts moving. Is an indication of **Rhus toxicodendron**. There is stretching and drawing in the limbs. With the fever there is dry teasing cough, external chill with internal heat, paroxysm of stretching and yawning, and frequently accompanied by urticaria. It is frequently indicated in typhoid fever. This is **Rhustox** fever.

There are distressing bone pains, with general soreness and periodicity. Restlessness, soreness of muscles and bones with changing periodicity. Chill is preceded by thirst, and great soreness and aching of bones. Perspiration relieves all pains except the headache. There is intense thirst but drinking causes vomiting. With the development of temperature it is necessary to examine skin for any eruption developing on it. The remedy is **Eupatorium perfoliatum**.

As the days of fever progress look for any rash developing. Rash developing on the first day of temperature may be Chicken pox or Dengue. Developing rash on the second day is Scarlatina and Erysepelas; Rash developing on the third day is small pox; Fourth day is Measles; Rubella develops from first day to fourth day, and Typhoid fever usually eighth day to tenth day. Each of these eruptions have special and distinctive characters together with day of its onset.

The patient experiences a onset of fever developing after a sudden change frcm hot or dry to damp weather, even develops catarrh in warm moist relaxing weather; is worse in cold damp weather and worse from fog. There is much muscular soreness, great prostration and headache, trembling and, therefore, wants to be held. Fever with stupor, dizziness, faintness, thirstlessness, prostration.This indicates **Gelsemium.** It is indicated in bilious remittant, malarial typhoid, cerebrospinal fevers and at the early stage of measles. It is initially indicated in the first week of typhoid where the patient feels sore and bruised all over as if he had been pounded — therefore dreads to move, has headache more than loss of muscular power. In such cases **Gelsemium** will modify the fever and the patient passes through comparatively milder symptoms.

There is an onset of fever after injury to the muscles,,drawing pains in the bones and periosteum, There is thirst with chill. The parts lain on are most affected, and patient keeps on changing positions. The face is hot and the body is cool. With the temperature rising high there is tendency of involvement of meninges. Becomes unconscious when spoken to but answers correctly. The sweat is sour, fetid and offensive. This bodyache continues even after the temperature comes down to normal. This is indicated in **Arnica.**

Arnica is complementary to and follows well after Aconite and complementary to Rhus tox and Hypericum. According to Hahnemann, Arnica is frequently indicated in cases treated with quinine, or abuse of quinine.

The progress of these simple fevers will get aborted within a week in a Psoric constitution and the subject would be symptom-free with indicated remedies. But if the constitution is Sycotic there is no remission and then they will start showing, some clues to the nature of their appearance and more deep acting remedies may be indicated.

As the temperature enters into the second week of its duration the early inflammatory picture and quick response of the body changes to something like toxaemia or septicaemia state. The picture changes from that fast and quick acting response of the system to slow but deep-acting ones, and deep acting drugs are indicated.

The temperature causes great weakness and anaemia and the paroxysms are fully developed, the three stages of chill, fever, sweat are fully marked. Preceding the chill there is violent thirst, and often violent temporal headache. There is an interval between the chill and fever but rarely in gastric disturbances. During fever there is generally thirst and sometimes unnatural hunger. The sweat is profuse and debilitating thirst during the pyrexia, great debility, ringing in the ears, feeling of emptiness in the stomach, and soreness in the stomach. This is **Cinchona officinalis** or **China.**

The fever has turned intermittent, chill beginning at about 10 a.m. with thirst, and drinking that does not relieve but profuse sweat relieves all symptoms. Throbbing frontal headache usually accompanies the chill and fever. In malarial intermittent fever there is profuse watery stool with great oppression of breath, coldness about the heart, and headache with great prostration. Sometimes the onset of paroxysm is accompanied by intense itching over the whole body and shaking chill. This picture resembles **Natrum muriaticum.**

3. ***Patient usually, a child, suffers from catarrh of the ocular, nasal and respiratory mucous membrane and by an eruption of minute elevated papules with fever and rash appearing on the fourth day. It may be MEASLES.***

After an incubation period of 10-12 days the symptoms start developing. At the commencement of the incubation there is a transient febrile catarrh, and a fleeting rash. There is a gradual development of fever with increase in catarrhal symptoms. During the first four days there is development of rash, usually on the late third day or the fourth day, catarrhal symptoms like sneezing, conjunctival inflammation, with short dry cough, tonsils get inflammed and koplik spots appear on the third day on the buccal mucosa around and in front of the parotid duct. But the most important point is that the child looks like a bundle of misery. The rash starts appearing behind the ears, along the margins of the forehead, temple and neck.

At this stage we are reminded of ***Aconite, Allium cepa, Euphrasia and Gelsemium.*** These remedies, when given at the right time, often abort the whole condition. But for some reason, if they do not, then at least they reduce intensity of the infection.

Bryonia alba is the first remedy that comes to mind. Normally when the rash is developing very slow or suddenly start receding or when the rash has not fully developed. The cough is dry, scraping of throat, and in fact represents the correct picture of measles.

Gelsemium: early morning sneezing and streaming colds are a strong indication of Gels. There is excessive weakness and trembling; the characteristic headache beginning in the occiput, and spreading over the whole head The skin is hot and dry, with eruptions developing, and this Gelsemium helps in bringing out the eruption.

Since both the drugs are slow-acting they will be required to be given on long-term basis till the eruption fully develops and then subsides. The course of the disease then changes for the better without leaving behind any complications.

Pulsatilla: has feverish hot body but the temperature is normal, used as a prophylactic for measles, there is chilliness without thirst, worse by warmth — the character of this drug. Ear trouble which is a common sequelae and complication of measles is corresponding to pulsatilla. Pulsatilla 3C is almost a prophylactic against measles. Mullien oil can be used as ear drops.

Morbillinum: a nosode, characterizes an attack of measles. It has fever, nasal and eye catarrh, nasal voice, rough cough, diffused bronchial cough, followed by macular eruption. As a prophylactic it is given to those who are likely to get exposed to infection and it is given in 30C twice or thrice daily. Belladonna given in 30C appears to heighten the effect. Only these two remedies can carry through the whole attack of the infection.

4. ***Patient, usually a child, develops an eruption of successive crops of limpid vesicles usually accompanying a slight elevation of fever, it is mostly a trivial disorder of childhood. It is accompanied by malaise, headache and backache and sometimes a prodromal scarlatiniform, morbilliform or urticarial rash, within 24 hours a characteristic rash appears. It is a case of CHICKEN POX or VARICELLA.***

The characteristic eruption is dark pink, slightly raised, ovoid or somewhat pyramidal papules which, in the course of few hours, become vesicular. The typical vesicle is at first a thin-walled translucent, unilocular, glistening bleb which contains a clear fluid, in the most superficial layer of the skin. After a day or so, this fluid is invaded by staphylococcus causing the fluid to become turbid. The vesicles in-between looses tension and dries into a scab. Within two weeks these scabs fall off leaving behind a pigmented scab. Pleomorphism is the character of this rash. The temperature rarely exceeds beyond 103° F . These scabs are very infectious and need to be disposed off by burning.

Antimonium Tartaricum is suited to children and old people, worn out and of hydrogenoid constitution. Eruptions are slow to develop, slow to recede with itching on the skin, eruptions leave a bluish mark, and the eruption are thick like pox-mark, copious cold clammy sweat, with great faintness.

Pulsatilla: has feverish hot body, commonly indicated in childhood fevers. Temperature is erratic. Child is chilly yet very averse to heat. Chilliness without thirst, cannot tolerate cold.

Rhustox: it has rheumatic constitution and is easily affected by getting wet or drenched in sweat or in rain. The onset of fever is with yawning, stretching, and aching of limbs, associated with dry teasing cough either before the chill develops or at beginning of the chill. The face is hot but the cheeks are cold. Occasionally there is urticaria. The very day there is temperature there is rash developing on the body which gets filled with fluid. These vesicles start increasing in number and the pleomorphism is present. The characteristic constitutional symptoms are present and tongue is coated alongwith its red triangular tip. This rash fully develops in four to six days and gradually starts receding over the next seven days with formation of scabs.

The pathogenesis of Ant Tart, Pulsatilla, Rhustox closely resemble that of Chicken pox.

5. ***Patient complains of sudden rise of temperature, chilly feeling, or a rigor followed by headache, aching eyeballs, and rapid rise of temperature. Excruciating backache, and joint pains follow, joints have particular swelling and redness. It is a case of DENGUE.***

In other words, this fever is called break-bone fever. This is a specific fever lasting not more than seven days. And onset is with rigor, chilly feelings, followed by headache and rapid rise of temperature even up to 105 °F. The tongue is furred and conjunctiva injected. Anorexia, vomiting, restless and insomnia may ensue. Often within two or three days the red rash appears on the skin. Initially there is tachycardia, but later becomes slow and then the temperature falls down on the third day. But gradually it starts rising again, and lasts for two or three days.

Eupatorium perf.: is a boon in those miasmatic districts, along the rivers, marshes etc. and is known as bone set because its prompt action to relieve the bone pains. There is typical chill preceded by thirst, with great soreness and aching of bones. Pain in bones as if broken. Burning heat, sweat relieves all symptoms, except the headache. Nausea, vomiting at the close of chill or hot stage, throbbing headache, knows the chill is coming because in spite of being thirsty cannot drink. The fever paroxysm usually commences in the morning,

Rhus toxicodendron: temperature starts with great restlessness, stiffness and soreness. Extremely chilly, with dry cough, inflammation of the eye, dilatation of the pupil, great restlessness worse by rest. But then the movement relieves his conditions.

6. *Patient develops sudden rise of fever, and rises in few hours to 102-104 °F, with severe headache, pain behind the eyes, shivering, anorexia, pains in the limbs and back. These are the characteristic features of INFLUENZA.*

There may be true bradycardia, and malaise and prostration are out of proportion to the temperature. Catarrh usually accompanies.

Arsenic alb: is wonderful winter remedy when influenza strikes. Apart from other symptoms of Arsenic alb., sneezing is characteristic. Thin nasal watery discharge, which excoriates the upper lip, and is accompanied by dull throbbing frontal headache.

Eupatorium perf.: has hoarseness worse in the morning and cough with extreme soreness in the chest, along the trachea. There is aching all over the body and the temperature creeps in at 7 a.m. to 9 a.m. and is preceded by headache and insatiable thirst, which rarely continues into fever.

Rhus tox: has typical influenza fever, the patient is restless, stiff, and sore. Chill with dry cough, and urticarial rash during heat. Chilly: worse by least covering. There is hoarseness of voice. Frequent changing of position for relief.

Influenzinum: it is a nosode Influenza. It is usually prescribed in 12C or 30C either in liquid or pill form. Usually ten pellets are dissolved in six ounces (170 ml) of water , a dessert spoon is as a dose. And may be repeated every two hours. It is claimed that latrge number of population is controlled.

General direction of Clarke is when there is beginning of cold that appears in the family, give Arsenic alb 3c thrice daily to all those who are not affected and give Influenzin 30c every one hour or two. It generally prevents the spread of the trouble and clears up the colds whether they are of influenza type or not. It is claimed to have effect on all types of influenza and their accompaniment like weakness and fatigue, influenza, encephalitis, enterocolitis of influenza etc.

Oscillococcinum a nosode was described by Joseph Roy in 1925, some oscillatory movements in the culture were detected in the germs and named the nosode as oscillococcinum. Dr. Pierre Schmidt says it is very useful in the beginning of Influenza as well as during convalescence. It is useful in all types of influenza especially in the early stages, bursting headache with muscular aches. Use the remedy in 200c every two to three hours or repeat only if necessary.

7. ***Patient comes with severe frontal headache, simple malaise and lassitude, mild bronchial cough, abdominal discomfort, anorexia, with pain and discomfort in the right iliac fossa, irregular bowels and constipation. If the patient comes a week later there is high continued fever. The temperature is characteristically rising in step ladder-like pattern, and there is slower pulse. The condition is TYPHOID FEVER.***

Typhoid fever is progressively developing disorder and, therefore, the indications of remedies will be different at different stages of the fever :

Gelsemium: at the onset when the patient seems to have taken cold and the picture starts developing very suddenly Gelsemium looks to be the remedy. It has the typical chill, running down the back, but thirst is absent. The pulse is slow, full and soft and compressible. Fever is associated with stupor, dizziness and faintness, and the patient is prostrated.

Nux vomica: is chilly and needs to cover in every stage, but the body is burning hot. Aching in the limbs, and back, and gastric symptoms. Chill with thirst and heat without thirst.

Arnica: is known for septic and traumatic fevers. It is useful in continuous and intermittent fevers. Thirst during chill. Must uncover but that chills. Fear at night, and on awakening, fear of crowd, and public places. Often goes into coma, muttering delirium but when spoken to answers correctly and relapses into delirious state. Whole body is sensitive and sore.

Bryonia and **Rhus tox** are again very important. Their symptoms are well-known.

As the time goes by and the remedies are not prescribed at the appropriate stage the picture changes into a toxaemic state or septicaemic state and the general picture of the patient changes.

The temperature continues to be at a higher level, and there is not much of diurnal remission but the pulse continues to be slow and dicrotic in proportion to temperature, blood pressure is lowered. There is eruption on the skin, spleen gets enlarged, lethargy becomes very marked, drowsiness deepens to semi-coma, occasionally there is diarrhoea, like pea soup, or yellow ochre, there is tympanitic distension of the abdomen. But this condition dramatically changes in the fourth week and the patient is on road to recovery. There may be apyrexial period but relapses are common.

Baptisia: there is generalized malaise as from severe illness, sore and bruised feeling. Chill is all-day long running up and down during the heat stage — the heat is all over the body.Dry skin, offensive and foetid sweat. During apyrexia there is sick, sore feeling all over the body and this fever is like that of Arnica, Arsenic and Gelsemium. In the third weeks gastric complaint, arise. Sensitive ileocoecal area. The most important mental symptom with the pyrexia is that the patient falls asleep while answering.

Phosphorus: as the patient enters the third week of temperature like Baptisia it also has gastric complications, rice watery stools, sago-like particles. The patient is sensitive to external impressions, light, noises and touch. There is chill every evening, without thirst and develops a ravenous hunger, and prefers ice-cold things. There are often respiratory and gastric complications.

Phosphoric acid: during the third week cerebral symptoms appear, regardless of the surroundings there is complete apathy, the sweat is profuse, exhausting, and there is thirst during the sweat stage.

Muriatic acid: great debility, with moaning unconsciousness, cold extremities. Patient slides down the bed automatically, there is great prostration.

Pyrogen: suited in conditions of septicaemia. Severe bone pains in the limb, with chill in the back as soon as the back touches the cold bed-sheet. The pulse is out of proportion to temperature abnormally rapid. The tongue is red, clean and like varnished.

The temperature with the right remedy will start coming down in a step-ladder like manner or lysis, and it takes time for the patient to come back to normal. It is our observation that the time taken for the patient to return to normal is much shorter than any other treatment. The general weakness that follows after the temperature has remitted, is also short. And the patient carries on normal activity in shortest possible time.

The incidence of classical typhoid has considerably reduced with the improvement of hygiene and general management. The latest diagnostic methods gives the physician an early indication and the physician takes appropriate steps. Therefore the temperature rarely goes beyond the fourth or the fifth day.

8. *A child, normally under the age of five, initially suffering from catarrh usually followed by paroxysmal attack of coughing succeeded by long noisy inspiration and usually followed by vomiting and fever is a case of* WHOOPING COUGH.

Please refer to the chapter on Respiratory diseases.

9. *A child starts with a moderate fever of 102 °F, with or without rigor, slow pulse, with headache, malaise, constipation and anorexia. Sore throat and stiffness of the neck and inflammatory swelling of one or both the parotid glands. The condition is MUMPS or PAROTITIS.*

Mercurius Iodat. Ruber. (Merc.Bin. Iod.) : it affects the lymphatic glands, throat but only on the left side. The fauces are dark red, and swallowing becomes painful. Sore throat — shifts from left to right. Tonsils and the adjoining glands are greatly swollen. The parotid gland on the left is painful with inadequate salivation. Stiffness of muscles and neck. There is intense shivering followed by fever and night sweats. Worse on empty swallowing.

Mercurius iod. flavus (Merc Proto iod) : sore throat goes from right to left and swelling begins at the right side. Sensation of lump worse on the right side. Constant inclination to swallow.

Lachesis: there is swelling on the parotid glands with purple-coloured throat seen from inside. Pain while swallowing liquids and hot drinks. Constrictive feeling better felt while eating. Heat on the vertex in flushes on waking and when falling asleep.

Baryta carb: takes cold easily with stitches and smarting pains. Submaxillary glands and tonsils are swollen, and can swallow liquids only.

Belladonna: effects are sudden and violent. Hot red skin, flushed face, dilated pupils, and throbbing carotids. Dryness of throat and water with aversion to water. Throat feels contracted, swallowing difficulty of liquids, therefore drinks in sips.

Pulsatilla: there is frequent inclination to clear throat, throat is dry and smarts on waking; scratchy and husky feeling in the throat. Painful drawing in left cheek-bone and jaw.

Parotidinum: is nosode and is used like a prophylactic against infection by mumps. Usually given in 6c or 30c, two to three times a day, in those exposed to the infection. It can be given in the disease condition every four hours, singly or alternated with the indicated remedy. It is also useful in post-mumps orchitis.

10. ***A child suffering from a gradual onset of fever over a day or two, with general listlessness, pallor, headache and vomiting. Soft and rapid pulse, sore throat and dysphagia with congestion of the throat. On examination of the throat reveals a thin membrane spreading to larynx and bronchi. A very diagnostic odour to the breath. The condition of DIPHTHERIA.***

Apis: Acts on the cellular tissue of the throat causing oedema, and produces inflammation with effusion.There is constricted stinging pain with swollen uvula, Diphtheria with early prostration, dirty membrane, sore throat, swallowing is painful but better by cold drinks. Thirstless during fever but thirst is during the chill.

Arsenic : High, hectic fever. But the body is cold as ice. There is complete exhaustion. Swollen throat, oedematous, constricted, burning and unable to swallow and everything swallowed appears to have lodged in oseophagus. Diphtheria membrane is dry and wrinkled. And there is aphonia.

Phytolacca : The throat is dark red and bluish red with much pain at the root of the tongue. There is pseudo-membranous exudate, greyish white, thick, tenaceous, yellowish mucus. The pains shoot in the ears with swallowing. Hot feeling as if a hot ball is placed in the throat. Burning worse by hot drinks.

Lac caninum : The throat is very sensitive to touch, painful on swallowing, and the pains extend to the ears. Tonsillitis and Diphtheria symptoms change repeatedly from side to side, shining glazed appearance of deposits, pearly white, or pure white porcelain, stiffness of the neck and tongue. Sore throat begins and ends with the menses. There is internal chilliness with external warmth. Exhaustive sweats after waking up in the morning.

Diphtherinum : The potencies of this nosode are prepared either from the Diphtheria bacteria or the membranes. These potencies are effective not only in the cases of Diphtheria but also in post-diphtheria paralysis.

Diphtherinum is useful as a prophylactic in Diphtheria and post-Diphtheria paralysis, and when anti-diphtheritic vaccination is used. It is adapted to patients prone to catarrhal disorders of respiratory organs, scrofulous individuals. In case of relapsing diphtheria, severe sore throats and inflamed tonsils with tendency to colds and bronchitis and palpitations. These are mostly the psoric or tubercular patients prone to catarrhal disoders of throat and respiratory mucous membrane. Patient is better from cold and drinking milk in sips. Better by heat and when in bed.

However, the use of Von Behring's antitoxin is a great advance and has proved a blessing to humanity.

11. *There is fever which is continuous or remittent type, and that goes on for some time and a typical periodic fever starts commencing during the midday with headaches and bodyaches, and pain in the limbs. These vague features have characteristic phases. The cold stage, lasting for half to two hours when the patient is lying in a curled up position, with blankets yet shivering. This is followed by hot stage where the blankets are discarded, and lasts for 4 to 5 hours, and perhaps vomiting and delirium may ensue. Then begins the sweat stage, which lasts for about two hours. This is MALARIAL FEVER.*

Malaria is an intermittent fever caused by four different types of parasites which infect the red blood corpuscles of man, and give rise to periodic paroxysms of fever, enlargement of spleen and anaemia. The transmission is by Anopheline mosquitoes.

Arsenic is one of the best remedies for intermittent fever and chill. Its periodicity comes every day, every third or fourth day, every fortnight, every six weeks, or even once a year. There is pronounced night aggravation, and restlessness. Worse nearing or after midnight; worse from cold and damp, better by warmth and prefers warm wraps. Externally cold but internally hot and burning. Sweat with great thirst, dyspnoea or exhaustion.

Cedron has regular paroxysm of fever, coming at the same hour, by chills in the back and limbs, or cold feet and hands. Burning heat in the hands, pulse is full and accelerated, and there is thirst for desire for warm water. Shivering and chill, with congestion in the head. Hand feet, nose, remain cold.

China officinalis has typical intermittent fever from marsh miasm — tertian or quartan type, chill and heat without thirst, thirst occurring either before or after chill and the chill is followed by long lasting heat with desire to uncover. Profuse and debilitating sweat follows. In apyrexial period the face is shallow, yellow, with enlarged spleen, loss of appetite. Periodicity is the leading characteristic both in fever and neuralgias, worse every other day.

Eupatorium perf.: Chill is preceded by thirst with great soreness, acihng bones as if broken, sweat relieves all the symptoms except headache. Vomiting of bile at close of chill, scanty sweat, nausea, knows his chill is coming because he cannot drink sufficient water. Fever paroxysm usually starts in the morning.

Natrum mur: has morning chill with thirst, chill between 9 a.m and 11 a.m.; although chilly is worse by sun/heat. Violent thirst increases with fever, coldness of the body. Marked continous chilliness, constipation, loss of appetite.

We have seen the typical remedies of intermittent fever where the pathogenesis coresponds with the intermittent fever. There are many remedies which resemble the intermittent fevers either partially or with characteristic symptoms. Repertory is the best source for this.

12. ***Patient, usually a child, complains of nasopharyngeal catarrh, intially with irregular fever, accompanied by fleeting joint pains, headache, vomiting and later skin rashes. Later the temperature is rarely above 102° to 104°F; these septicaemic symptoms are either succeeded or accompanied by irritating intracranial inflammations, such as severe headaches, vomiting, photophobia, restlessness, drowsiness and delirium retraction of the head often noticed. The condition most probably CEREBRO-SPINAL FEVER.***

This is sporadic or appears in epidemics in infants and children usually in spring and winter. It is infectious. It spreads through droplet infection. Although developed countries this has become rare but in over-populated countries like ours it is still a common disorder. Isolation is best. And the patient should be nursed in dark room. Initial diagnostic lumbar puncture is advised.

Apis mel. Burning heat, afternoon chill with thirst, worse on motion and heat. Sleeps after the fever paroxysm, brain feels very tired, dull and heavy sensation in the occiput, as from a blow, sudden stabbing in the head. Sharp shrieks, bores the head into the pillow, and screams out. Rolling of the head from side to side, boring the head backwards into the pillow.

Belladonna : develops throbbing and hammering headaches, worse by motion and worse in the temples by light, noise, jar or lying down. Heat, burning, redness are the three characteristics of Belladonna. High fever with delirium but there is no thirst with fever.

Gelsemium : great prostration and headache, chill with aching and languor, chills up and down the spine, nervous chills and total lack of thirst. The headache starts in the occiput, and spreads over the front of the head.

Opium: generally low temperature, with inclination to stupor. Hot sweaty and drowsy. With cold limbs. Heat extending over the body, with hot perspiration, sweat without relief. Pulse is slow but full snoring respiration.

Diet

The diet in fever should mainly consist of nourishing fluids. Boiled water, barley water with or without lemonade, glucose water, lemon barley water. Fruit juices can be given in-between. Diluted milk is permitted.

Soft cooked rice with plenty of rice water can be given.

'Khichdi' — a combination of lentil and rice — well cooked with salt to taste, about 4 tablespoons can be given.

Boiled egg with pepper and salt can be given.

Nowadays many proprietary predigested food products are available. The contents are printed on it, also contents are mentioned.

Usually with fever over a period and the movements being reduced, the bowels tend to constipate. Movement of the bowels must be encouraged by give warm drinks

2 RESPIRATORY SYSTEM

- Cardinal symptoms of respiratory diseases
- Upper respiratory infections — Differential therapeutics
- Lower Respiratory infections — Differential therapeutics
- Investigations
- Management

We have witnessed over the last 50 years or so a tremendous boost in the development of industrialization, both in the rural and urban areas, causing increased risk of pollution. Although many rules and laws have been framed to curb the spread of the menace it has not been effectively checked. This has caused an increase in respiratory sufferings. Modernization and international travel have increased the fear of spread of communicable diseases. Smoking has become a status symbol in the young adults, it has become sign of maturity! All these changes have caused increase in the respiratory disorders and they are gradually spreading out of proportions.

In addition to this, hyper-sensitization to various allergens — both chemical as well as plants — contribute to this malady. Modernization and changed life style has reduced the time for recreation and exercise. All these have taken a big toll on the health status of our society.

Cardinal Symptoms of Respiratory Diseases

Cardinal symptoms of respiratory disorders are *(1) Cough, (2) Breathlessness, (3) Expectoration, and, at times (4) Pain in the chest and Haemoptysis.*

1. Cough can be dry or accompanied by expectoration. If dry, it can be simple congestion of the throat or larynx, or early pleurisy, or some pulmonary disorder or some source of reflex irritation. A night cough can be because of chronic congestion of the pharynx. The long barking or nervous cough can be of hysteria. A short suppressed cough of pleurisy is almost diagnostic. Brassy cough is present with

aneurysm and other mediastinal tumours. The reflex coughs are due to irritation in the area of the vagus nerves, like gastro-intestinal disorders, worms in the intestine, pericarditis, ear trouble, irritation of the diaphragm by subphrenic or liver abscesses.

2. In fact, breathlessness is related more with the cardiac problems. Any nasal or naso-pharyngeal catarrh produces sniffing and nasal bubbling. When this is attended by considerable wheezing in the chest, it is characteristic of bronchitis. Stridulous respiration is caused by obstruction or pressure on trachea or the larynx. Continuous dyspnoea may be present in a gross disease of the chest or with emphysema.

3. Recurring wheezing cough is accompanied by expectoration, in asthma, and/or carcinoma of the bronchii. Paroxysms of cough followed by vomiting is present in whooping cough, and advanced phthisis. Purulent cough is in bronchiectasis, irritable and mainly dry cough is in early phthisis.

4. Pain in the chest is usually associated with affections of the pleura. Sharp and cutting pain on one side is in pleurisy, pneumonia. A soreness behind the sternum can be because of tracheitis and bronchitis. Sudden severe pain followed by considerable pulmonary distress and general collapse occurs in the onset of pneumothorax. Cancer of the lungs, mediastinal tumours can also give pain in the chest. Haemoptysis means spitting of the blood and, in fact, it is usually restricted to the lower respiratory tract, larynx, trachea, bronchi or lungs. This bleeding can be from streaks of blood mixed with sputum to profuse haemorrhage.

For the sake of convenience of our study we may group the complaints of these patients in two groups. One, the complaints arising in the upper respiratory organs; and, two, in the lower respiratory organs.

1. ***The patient complains of tiredness, slight elevated temperature, malaise, a sore nose and pharynx. Profuse watery nasal discharge and sneezing; eventually turning thick and muco-purulent.The condition may be ACUTE CORYZA OR COMMON COLD.***

This is a highly infectious illness comprising a mild systemic upset but having prominent nasal symptoms, infection can occur from close personal contact or from droplets. The incidence of infection is high in the early stages of the infection and the spread is facilitated by overcrowding and poor ventilation system. The condition can persist up to a week. Psoric and Pseudo-Psoric constitutions are more susceptible to this infection.

In a very early stage when the infection has just started showing its effects.

Saponaria: is a very useful remedy in the treatment of acute colds, coryza, sore throat, it often helps to break the cold.

Aconite: has sudden onset from exposure to cold, cold dry northern winds. Fluent coryza, frequent sneezing, inflammation of the throat with high fever, spasmodic cough, tightness and oppression of the chest, and stitches in the chest while breathing. Great anxiety, restless, anxious and frightened expression.

Allium cepa: has coryza, steaming eyes and nose, with headache, frequent sneezing, profuse acrid discharge from nose. Tickling in larynx — Catarrhal laryngitis.

Cough from inhaling cold air. Although it stops the catarrh quickly it may drive the trouble to the chest. Phosphorus corrects this action.

Euphrasia: is similar to Allium cepa but here we have excoriating lachrymation but bland nasal discharge.

Arsenic album: always takes colds in the nose, and sneezes from every change in the weather. Thin watery discharge from the nose, excoriating the upper lip, while the nose is stuffed up all the time: Violent spasmodic sneezing: Itching, burning and watering of the eyes: Chilly, with burning relieved by heat. Restless; Anxious; Thirsty.

Gelsemium: cold develops several days after exposure, usually in winters. Catarrh is hot, watery, excoriating, in warm moist and relaxing weather. Teasing and tickling cough better near the fire; tiredness of the whole body; Chill up and down the back: Thirstless.

Ammonium carbonicum: is particularly suited to winter catarrh. The nose is stopped at night, worse at 3 to 4 a.m., Cough dry, tickling, with hoarseness. Nostrils are sore and raw, there is stoppage of one nostril in Ammon mur.

Dulcamara: cold develops in cold wet weather, or from getting wet, or chilled when heated. Or from sudden changes in the atmosphere from hot to cold. Dry coryza, sore throat, stiff neck, worse in open air: Coryza more fluent in the warmth of the house and less fluent in the cold air (Nux). Eyes become red and sore with every cold, Nose gets stuffed with cold, rain.

Kali iodatum: cold develops from every exposure to damp weather: Red nose, acrid nasal discharge, eyes smart and lachrymate, Catarrhal inflammation of the frontal sinuses, eyes, throat, and chest. Nasal voice; violent thirst; Alternate heat and chill.

Natrum muriaticum: has catarrh, thin watery, at times thick like white of an egg: Paroxysms of sneezing. Worse exposure to fresh air, Cough with headache, Urine spurts while coughing, Loves salt.

Sabadilla: spasmodic sneezing with running nose. Copious watery nasal discharge, fluent coryza. Worse on from smelling of flowers, oversensitiveness to odours. Dry itching in the nose, rubs and picks at the nose. One or the other nostril is stuffed up; cannot tolerate the smell of garlic.

2. ***The patient complains of tiredness, very slight fever, malaise and sore nose with thin watery discharge associated with headache and facial pain and tenderness. The condition is SINUSITIS.***

It often complicates the upper respiratory infection, e.g Coryza or Allergic Rhinitis.

It is difficult to differentiate sinusitis from the symptoms of common cold. The remedial treatment is the same as in case of common cold.

Kali bichromicum: has, in addition to the other symptoms of cold, pain at the root of the nose, coryza with obstruction of the nose, violent sneezing and thick slimy discharge. Chronic inflammation of the frontal sinus.

Natrum arsenicosum: has post-nasal dripping of thick bland yellow mucus. There is obstruction of nose which is followed by headache. It facilitates the termination of cold *Cartier;* the headache is aggravated by pressure and tobacco smoke.

Nux vomica: gets the nose stuffed after exposure to dry cold atmosphere, worse in warm room. The coryza is fluent during the daytime but nose is stuffed up at night and outdoors; or it alternates between nostrils although there is discharge, the nose feels stuffed up.

Hydrastis canadensis: sinusitis develops after coryza, with post-nasal dripping. Thick tenacious yellow secretion. Coryza, excoriating, burning, smarting and rawness. Nose bleed with burning rawness, followed by itching, constant discharge of thick white mucus.

Mercurius: sinusitis, and colds, acrid discharge but too thick to run down the lips, worse in warm room. Frequent sneezing with coryza, sneezing in sunshine. Nostrils are raw and ulcerated. Swelling of the nasal bones and decay with greenish fetid ulceration.

Thuja: chronic catarrh, thick yellow green mucus. Bloody scabs or briny odour in the nose. This is a chronic nasal infection — yellow green discharge. Dryness of the nasal cavities.

Silicea: frothy nasal discharge, nose-bleed, perforation of the septum, Dry hard crusts from bleeding when loosened. Sneezing in the morning, itching at the tip of the nose. Obstinate cold with ear affection. Loss of smell.

Pulsatilla: catarrh, loss of smell, coryza is better going out in the open. Abundant yellow mucus in the morning, pressing pain at the root of the nose.

3. ***The patient complains of nasal irritation, sneezing and rhinorrhoea or blockage, associated with itching of the eyes and soft palate or even ears for an hour or so for most of the days. This condition is RHINITIS, and if it is present throughout the year it is called PERENNIAL RHINITIS.***

When it is limited for a particular period of the year, it is called SEASONAL RHINITIS.

The seasonal rhinitis is due to various pollutants that pervade the atmosphere from time to time such as pollens of the trees, grass, moulds that grow on the cultivated plants and also those moulds which grow on the decaying plant material such as compost, piles of leaves etc.

The perennial rhinitis rarely have symptoms that affect the eyes or throat. The symptoms are either sneezing and watery nose or just the blocking of the nose. The major cause of this is the faecal matter of the house, dust mite that nourishes on the desquamated human skin scales and are found in abundance in the human bedding, industrial dust and vapour, fumes, cigarette smoke, perfumes, washing powders; household detergents are not real culprits but since the nose of the perennial rhinitis is very sensitive, it becomes more reactive to non-specific stimuli as well.

Arsenic album: is one of the major remedies that satisfies all the symptoms of these varieties of rhinitis. Must have other characteristics of the drug.

Arum triphyllum: has sore nostrils, acrid and excoriating thin discharge, obstructed nose, boring in the nose, and constant picking at the nose till it bleeds.

Ambrosia: has profuse lachrymation and intolerable itching of the eyelids, stuffed nose and chest: must sit up to breathe comfortably, wakes up with sudden pertussis-like cough, worse in the evening, till midnight. Tincture in 3rd potency 10 drops in water during and after the attack usually helps.

Rosa damascena: is useful in the beginning of the attack, usually when there is involvement of the eustachian tube.

Wyethia: has a very characteristic symptom of itching of the soft palate — follicular pharyngitis — Kent used this as a prophylactic in hay fever. Tough ropy saliva, pain in the left ovary shooting down to the knee.

Sinapis nigra: is indicated when the nasal mucosa is dry and hot and there is no discharge, the symptoms are worse in the afternoon and evening. One nostril blocked, or both alternately stopped.

Sabadilla: is extremely sensitive to cold and is chilly, has violent and spasmodic sneezing and lachrymation, while going to the open air. Coryza is associated with severe frontal pains with redness of the eye.

4. ***Patient complains of nasal obstruction, loss of smell and taste. Lodged in the nose are smooth, semi-translucent glistening mucous bodies attached to the nasal wall with a relatively small slender pedicle. The condition is NASAL POLYP.***

It is mostly the Sycotic or Tubercular trait.

Calcarea Carb: is constitutionally close to its pathogenesis. These are children who are inclined to grow fat, and who take cold with the slightest change in weather. Have offensive smell in the nose but they do not have sense of smell, Bleeding. Then the remedy to think of is Phosphorus.

Sanguinaria nitricum: has profuse watery mucus discharge from the nostrils and burning.

Thuja: has enlarged turbinates, nostrils are plugged with thick yellow bloody mucus. Thuja has green chronic nasal catarrh with chronic sinus infection. It is remedy for self-exuberant fungoid tissue polyps, or condylomata, or warts.

Teucrium marum varum: has constant sense of crawling in the nose, catarrhal condition of both anterior and posterior nostrils, discharge of large irregular clinkers crawling in nostrils and, at times, stoppage of nostrils with coryza.

Lemna minor: Acts primarily upon the nostrils, develops these nasal polyps mostly in the wet weather, putrid post-nasal discharges but having loss of smell. With swollen turbinates. Atrophic rhinitis. Even develops asthma due to obstruction of the nostrils. Pain from nostril to the ear like string. Calcarea follows well.

5. ***Patient complains of a slight discomfort in swallowing, a dry throat, tickling and hawking cough. This haiss followed after a mild febrile catarrh. The condition is ACUTE PHARYNGITIS.***

Majority of these cases are due to viral infection and they run for 4-5 days. At times this acute pharyngitis extends to cause conjunctivitis, cervical adenitis, and in the lower respiratory tract extends to laryngitis, tracheitis, bronchitis and sometimes into pneumonia. Often this is accompanied with temperature. Another variety is due to influenza viruses with many constitutional symptoms like body-aches and sweating are produced.

Kali bichromicum: is indicated in follicular pharyngitis where the follicles of the throat get hypertrophied and look like tubercles on the pharyngeal wall. It discharges white offensive cheesy material and is attended by dryess in the throat, with accumulation of tenacious mucus.

Hepar sulph: has yellow tenacious mucus, sensation as if splinters or plug in the throat on swallowing: stitches in the throat extending up to the ears when swallowing. Hoarseness with loss of voice.

Ignatia: has plug-like sensation in the throat, with a tendency to choke. Stitches in the throat when not swallowing.

Chimaphila maculata: has swollen tonsils, and tensive pain in the throat on swallowing.

6. ***Child has difficulty in breathing through nose during the day, and, therefore, persistently breathes through open mouth. The voice develops a nasal twang, often accompanies the enlargement of tonsils. The case is NASOPHARYNGEAL ADENOIDS.***

The hypertrophied mass of lymphoid tissue constituting adenoids may fill the whole nasopharynx. They appear mostly in children and may spontaneously disappear as they grow. There is often an early morning sneezing and nasal obstruction may get worse in the afternoon. Often these children are susceptible to classroom dust.

Agraphis nutansis: the first and foremost remedy. Has obstruction of nasal passage with catarrhal condition, often deafness. Enlarged tonsils are associated with this. Lower potency is often suitable.

Calcarea Iod: is useful in scrofulous affections, especially in enlarged glands, tonsils and adenoids etc.

Baryta carb : submaxillary glands and tonsils are swollen, catches cold easily with stitches and smarting pains. Suppurating tonsils from cold. Tendency to enlargement of the glands.

7. ***Child complains of sore throat, and on swallowing there is severe pain. Heavily furred tongue, enlarged cervical glands. The temperature is 101- 104° F with mild rigor. The condition is ACUTE TONSILLITIS.***

Tonsillitis is often a forerunner of number of severe constitutional diseases such as scarlet fever, measles, rheumatic fever, acute nephritis, septicaemia, or acute mastoiditis. Substance of tonsils look red and swollen and inflamed. There are two varieties of these inflammations. One: Acute Parenchymatous tonsillitis, and the other: Follicular tonsillitis. Symptoms are same in both the cases. Streptococcus haemolyticus is the commonest pathogenic organism. Although S.aureus or S. viridance may also be the exciting causes. Whatever is the causative organism, the expression of signs and symptoms decide the remedy.

Belladonna: Is the first rank remedy. Typically an anti-psoric remedy. Angry looking dry and glazed look of the tonsils, mostly the right-sided tonsil is affected. Throbbing and congested pain. Swallowing, difficulty, with sensation of constriction in the throat.

Mercurius solubilis: there is constant desire to swallow, sticking into the ear. Pus points, sore, and burning pains in the throat: Loss of voice. Offensive odour in the mouth, feels better on sipping warm water.

Merc Bin Iod (Mercurius iodatum ruber): has particularly the left tonsillar infection and other symptoms of Mercurius are the same.

Merc Proto. Iod (Mercurius Iodatum flavous) : has the right-sided affection.

Hepar sulphuris: has splinter-like pains in the throat on swallowing. There is impending suppuration. Hoarseness with loss of voice. Generally a chilly patient.

Phytolacca: has dark bluish-red tonsils with pain at the root of the tongue. Sensation of lump in the throat. The throat feels rough, narrow and hot with swollen tonsils, pain shoots up to the ear on swallowing. Cannot swallow anything hot.

Lachesis: has livid and purple-coloured sore throat, worse on the left side, more painful on swallowing liquids. Pain extends up to the ear. Choking sensation at the neck and needs loose collar or neck-band, pain is aggravated by hot drinks.

Lac caninum: has a sensitive throat to touch which keeps on changing sides from left to right .Shining glazed or porcelain white surface of the tonsils. Starts at the beginning of the menses and ends with menses. Cough is caused by tickling sensation in throat.

Lycopodium: beginning of the sore throat is on the right side. Ulceration of the tonsils are worse by cold drinks.

Silicea: has a peculiar pain, pricking sensation in the tonsil; enlargement of parotid glands. Tonsils are suppurating and swollen. Develops very slowly.

Baryta carb: submaxillary glands and tonsils are swollen, takes cold easily with stitches and smarting pain, tonsils suppurate with taking cold everytime.

One has to remember that if these attacks of tonsils are very frequent — when an attack runs into another which do not give any respite to the patient from pain, fever, etc., then one should seriously think of surgical intervention to avoid further complications.

8. ***The patient reports with sudden illness that starts with fever, shivering and generalized aching in the limbs. This is also associated with severe headache, soreness of the throat and persistent dry cough. The patient is probably suffering from INFLUENZA.***

Aconite: has sudden onset of fever with chilliness and throbbing pulse, and great restlessness; the cause is often from anxiety, suppressed perspiration or exposure to dry cold winds.

Gelsemium: has heaviness and tiredness of the body and limbs, chill in the back, bursting headache from neck, over head to eyes and forehead, relieved by copious urination; but is always thirstless.

Eupatorium perf.: has intense aching limbs, as if bones were breaking. Cannot move for the fear of pain. Shivering and chill in the back that begins by 7 to 9 a.m. There may be vomiting of bile like that in the case of break-bone fever "dengue".

Bryonia: is indicated when the fever sets in on getting suddenly chilled after getting heated; wants to lie down still and needs to be left alone; the tongue is coated white with thirst for water or much cold fluids. The pains are better by pressure but worse by movements.

Rhus tox: has bruised lame and painful limbs on attempt to move but pass off as there is continued movement till he becomes tired when the pains appear again. Illness may start with dampness and getting wet while perspiring.

Pyrogen: has agonising pain in the lower limbs and the lumbar region, thigh muscles, that makes to remain still for a moment. Extremely chilly, no fire can give warmth. There is creeping chill in the back with thumping in the heart; the tongue has clean varnished look, and the pulse is out of proportion to fever.

Baptisia: has a sudden onset that runs rapidly to stupid typhoid state. Has besotted appearance, red but dull. Comatose and drops asleep while answering the question. There is sudden attack of violent diarrhoea, and vomiting associated with great prostration. It is often termed as "gastric flu".

(Also see Chapter 1 Pyrexia)

9. ***Patient comes with a history of irritating, unproductive cough, with discomfort behind the sternum, associated with tightness, shortness of breath and wheezing for two to three days. Cough, he says, has gradually become productive with greenish-yellow sputum and has mild fever. This is a case of ACUTE BRONCHITIS.***

On auscultation one finds an occasional crackle with wheeze and blood examination shows neutrophilic leucocytosis.

In an otherwise healthy person, without the patient being seriously ill, the whole episode can improve within 4-8 days. It is either because of bacterial or viral infection, from nasal sinuses or throat. Or this attack can be complication of measles, whooping cough etc. and inhalation of dust, gases like SO_2 or pollens or organic dust.

Aconite: is one of the first remedies that one thinks of in a case of acute bronchitis. That hoarse dry croupy cough, short and hacking, worse at night, provided the case is presented to the physician at the very onset of the illness. Remember, Aconite has a very short action time and if the time passes by the case shifts to Bryonia.

Bryonia: is indicated after the primary phase of Aconite is over and it fits into the disease description made above. In addition to that there is bursting pain in the head every time he coughs. This cough is worse after a meal and the cough may end into a vomit. To avoid the stitching pain in the chest he holds the sides while he coughs. At times little tenacious blood-streaked sputum is raised.

Kali bichromicum: has that hoarse voice, metallic, hacking cough worse in the evening, the pain is felt more at the bifurcation of the trachea on coughing from mid-sternum to the back. Thickly coated tongue and loathing of food is another characteristic.

Ipecacuanha: has an action on the pneumogastric nerve producing spasmodic irritation in the chest and stomach. Patient, often a child, coughs, gags, suffocates with a coarse rattling. Nausea is a constant accompaniment. There is clean tongue and patient is thirstless.

Convalescent stage is important. Patient may be allowed to sit up in bed, about four days after the subsidence of cough and expectoration. He should be asked to take 2-4 weeks' of rest before resuming work. Exposure can cause relapse. Change of air and deep breathing exercises should be advised.

10. ***The patient complains of sharp pain the chest on inspiration, has a short dry cough, with a moderately elevated temperature: on auscultation friction sounds are heard. The disease is DRY PLEURISY.***

Dry pleurisy is an inflammation of pleura without effusion. But there is a tendency to develop effusion and adhesions. The most obvious symptom is pain described as sharp stabbing, stitch-like or knife-like pain. This gives that characteristic 'catch' during inspiration. All other actions like laughing, yawning, coughing aggravate this pain. There is no breathlessness but shortness of breath due to fear of pain.

Aconite: is one of the most important remedy. Pleurisy arises from exposure to cold, sudden suppression of perspiration with distinct temperature. It has its characteristic mental restlessness with fear and dry short, hacking cough, worse at night usually after midnight. Everytime he coughs there is stitching in the chest. Jahr says that the whole trouble can be removed like magic with Aconite 30 given every two or three hours.

Bryonia: Dry hacking cough from irritation to the upper trachea, worse at night, after eating or drinking must sit up. Difficult quick respiration — worse from every movement — causes stitching pain in the chest. Bryonia invariably follows Aconite, when it has not completed its action or failed to control the march of the disease.

Ranunculus bulbosus: Another remedy that has soreness and bruised feeling of the chest right from sternum, ribs, intercostal spaces, to both the hypochondria. There is chilliness in the chest while walking in the open air. Breathing is short and oppressed with acute stabbing pain in the chest. The pulse is very rapid.

Kali Carb: dry hard cough around 3 a.m. with stitching pains in the chest . The entire chest is sensitive. Cutting pain in the chest that is aggravated lying on the right side. Bryonia has pain in the chest, mostly on movement, but unlike Bryonia in Kali Carb, it is independent of respiration.

11. ***The patient, a child, has paroxysms of coughing which terminates into a whoop and frequently in vomiting; there is some fever but only sign in the lung are those of little bronchial catarrh. The disease is WHOOPING COUGH (PERTUSSIS).***

Drosera rotundifolia: accredited by *Hahnemann* as the principle remedy for whooping cough. The cough is dry, irritating and spasmodic and the paroxysms follow each other rapidly. Can scarcely breath and chokes. The cough is deep and hoarse, worse after midnight. *Hahnemann* advises one single dose of 30 potency and to wait till the symptoms subside; but our experience is that one needs repeated doses in the present-day context.

Dr. Bayes advises fractional doses of mother tincture after every fit of paroxysm. But it is observed that in any manner you prescribe this is undoubtedly a very effective remedy against Whooping cough. Should the patient take cold during convalescence and the cough returns, Aconite and Ipecacuanha should be resumed.

Corallium rubrum: in 12th potency is suggested by Hartmann, it works a beneficial adjunct to Drosera. There is a dry, spasmodic suffocative cough with great sensitiveness to air passages and feels cold on inspiration.

Belladonna: as a remedy for catarrhal stage of whooping cough according to Bharr.

Cuprum metallicum: for the spasmodic stage. In case of Belladonna there is short tickling but dry cough with pain in the stomach before an attack, worse at night. In Cuprum the cough has a gurgling noise, better by drinking cold water. Suffocative attacks are worse at 3 a.m.

Pertussinum (Coqueluchin): was introduced as a nosode by John H Clarke — taken from the glairy and stringy mucus containing the virus of the whooping cough.— for whooping and spasmodic coughs.

12. ***The patient complains of the onset of a dry cough with malaise, and moderate fever, accompanied by pain in the chest that reduces gradually with passage of time; followed by sudden rise of fever to 103° -104°F mild rigor. On examination, the lower part of the chest is dull on one side, and over this area the vocal Fremitus and Resonance are Diminished or absent. The disease is PLEURISY WITH EFFUSION.***

Tuberculosis is by far the most common cause of sudden pleural effusion in young adults. Pseudo Psoric-constitutions are more susceptible.

One must observe the physical signs : Diminished movement of the chest wall or fullness or bulging of the chest wall; Impaired percussion note: Bronchial breathing and bronchophony: aegophony: Diminished air entry and diminished movement of the chest wall and of vocal resonance. Radiology of the chest will show uniform opaque area fading into normal lung markings, and, if the fluid is less, then the costophrenic angles will show obliteration.

Bryonia: still stands very high with that malaise, fever and pain in the right side of the chest. This will initially cover the inflammatory phase of the serous membrane.

Apis: becomes indicated when effusion sets in. Short dry cough, with a sense of suffocation, breathing becomes hurried and difficult, stinging pain in lower chest. Dropsical effusion of serous tissue is the characteristic pathological state of Apis. Patient is thirstless, and has burning and stinging sensation in the chest. Instead of using Apis, Jousset uses Cantheris.

Cantheris: there is intense dyspnoea; palpitations; and frequent dry cough. This needs to be repeated for long as he says the pleurisy with effusion is a very slow developing condition.

Phosphorus: can be easily identified by the typical burning spots in the chest, stitching in the left upper chest, dry cough. Congestion in the chest is aggravated by drinking cold water.

Sulphur: has sharp stitching pains through the left lung to the back, worse lying on the back and worse from least movement. Sulphur is also useful in such cases where we find recovery is either slow or not taking place in spite of well-chosen remedies, particularly when there is well marked pleuritic effusion.

When this pleuritic effusion undergoes purulent metamorphosis and empyema is present the scope of homoeopathy needs to be reassessed. Often evacuating the fluid by aspiration will be more judicious. Bahr recommends here **Mercurius** and **Hepar Sulphuris** for promotion of absorption.

Silicea: is a better choice since its absorption properties and prevention of fresh formation are better although the recovery is slow.

13. ***The patient is suddenly taken ill, with shivering attack or rigor: the temperature rises rapidly to 102° - 104° F with dry cough often with pleuritic pain. Sputum is rusty, signs of consolidation at the base of the lung. The_disease is ACUTE LOBAR PNEUMONIA.***

Lobar pneumonia has marked constitutional symptoms like shivering, rigor, headache, backache and high temperature. The face is flushed, anxious and little cyanosed. The urine is scanty and concentrated.

Aconite: a very characteristic history will be given of sudden onset, outdoor exposure to cold weather, and followed by temperature the same evening. High temperature with excitement, restlessness and acute anxiety. Full and bounding pulse, flushed face, hot and dry skin, dry mouth and intense thirst for cold water. The pupils are contracted, and, in spite of the hot and dry and flushed skin, the extremities are cold. Starts developing stabbing pain in the left chest, cannot lie on that side and likes to sleep on the back, propped-up. Brings on red strained sputum very little at a time. The pathogenesis of Aconite lasts mostly for 36 hours. There is no suggestion or indication of Aconite thereafter.

Ferrum Phos: is a quieter personality, takes a little longer to develop the picture than Aconite. Unlike Aconite, it will have a localized malar flush, has a disturbing cough, indisposed to talk. In both the cases the pulse rate and rhythm is same. Definitely chilly patient, sensitive to cold air and cough is aggravated by draught of cold air. Right side is more affected. The symptoms are aggravated usually in the morning whereas Aconite is aggravated in the evening.

Belladonna: has a very similar expression and the course like that of Aconite. But unlike Aconite it has bright red face, generalized blush over the whole skin, and the surface very hot to touch. There is intense excitement to the extent that it is difficult to keep the child in bed — almost impossible to control. Pupils are widely dilated, and hence an intense photophobia. But is afraid of dark and needs a light in the room — as long as it does not shine in their eyes they are fine. The tongue is typically strawberry. Intense, congestive, throbbing headache.

Ipecacuanha: can be considered in children, when the whole episode begins with vomiting. The onset here is slightly slower, with lack of appetite, gloomy, feeling sick, and a hot sweaty face. At the commencement there is bright red blood in the sputum. And severe sneezing attacks. In frank pneumonia, the tongue is clean but in case of bronchopneumonia the tongue is heavily coated but thirst is not present.Once the first 24 hours are over the excitement phase of the disease process is over and you may see different remedies.

The excitement dies down and the whole picture takes a very slow pace. One will find that the patient wakes up with a very dull face and drowsy look, heavy eyes and dullness over the eyebrows — **Bryonia** is indicated. The tongue is thickly coated with bitterness, and thirst for large quantity of water. He dislikes being disturbed and wants to lie down very quietly. There is often delirium and there they show the uncertainty of mind. They want to go home even if they are at home, they worry about their business, and think that they are still at their work. Initially the cough is non-productive but later it is very irritating and streak of redness in the sputum. Slightest movement hurts them. They are hot patients.

Phosphorus: pneumonia develops rather faster than Bryonia. An overworked and tired patient has got himself exposed to cold weather, feels an acute sense of oppression or tightness in the chest, same night develops a dry cough, with little hoarseness, or even actual loss of voice; develops a catchy respiration and the breathing becomes difficult; this is accompanied by burning in the chest. Extremely thirsty and desire cold water. They like to be propped up but with head tilted low back with chin tilted up. They are chilly patients, any draught of air aggravates but they still like to drink cold water! Cannot stay alone and want some physical contact.

There is not much of a difference in the Veratrum viridie patient from that of Phosphorus except that the V.viridie complains of intense pulsation as if pounding. There may be violence very early in the case with all sorts of obsessions. This is close to Belladonna but the face is not flushed and red but is very livid with beads of sweat. Profuse perspiration all over the body. He is intensely thirsty and anything that he drinks tastes very sweet. Eyes will show wide dilated pupils with intense photophobia.

Chelidonium: is another remedy that one should consider. In fact, Bryonia and Chelidonium have a very close resemblance. Grand difference between them is in terms of thirst and pain. Chelidonium desires warm drinks whereas Bryonia wants cold drinks. Although the remedies are both right-sided, the pains in Chelidonium are in front of the chest travelling towards the back whereas in Bryonia the pains are in the axilla travelling to the back. Bryonia wants to lie on the affected side but Chelidonium wants to sit up and lean forward.

It is always advisable to prescribe medium potencies at a regular interval of two hours and wait to see the changes. If one is very sure then high potency also can be prescribed at two or three hour intervals.

In cases of virulent pneumonia, which are often in winters, the onset, though slow, develop with astonishing rapidity. The virulence of the disease causes cerebral congestion resulting into dullness of mind and state of confusion.

The typical **Baptisia** mind prevails on thinking, speech and response. All are slow and are drowsy but restless. Their looks cyanosed with puffy face. They develop a very damp sweat that has unpleasant odour. The oppression in the chest gets aggravated on lying down. In short, it is more a toxic picture of Bryonia.

Pyrogen: pneumonia are more rapid than Baptisia and have a very flushed face, are loquacious, impatient, and they talk very fast. The temperature and pulse are characteristic but they are out of proportion to each other. The Pyrogen tongue is red, shining and varnished-like, unlike Baptisia. There are waves of heat that are followed by waves of shivering. Pyrogen has one more characteristic — at the onset of the pneumonia there is pain in the legs that spread upwards.

Lachesis: pneumonia, there is surging headache with every cough and a characteristic choking sensation at the throat and oppression at the chest with stabbing pain which is not better by pressure.

Mercury: will be another remedy that will come into the reckoning in the later part of winter. With the other characteristics of the remedy there will be swing in temperature with the instability to heat and cold. The cough tends to come in double paroxysms.

Hepar sulph: are extremely sensitive to cold, must cover with blanket till the neck and always wants the room to be hot .There are two main features of Hepar sulph in Pneumonia — one is aphthous ulcers spread out in the mouth but the patient prefers highly tasty drinks and food. And the other is — extreme weakness in the chest and acute stabbing pain in the chest which aggravate on lying on the affected side.

Rhus tox: is another chilly drug that is useful in pneumonia. Usually the story is that the patient on an outing has been soaked in rain and then got exposed to cold damp atmosphere. It will have all the other characteristics of the remedy.

In later stages of pneumonia or — where one has not seen the case in its earlier stages or a case that is not resolving well — there are some remedies that will help.

Antimonium tartaricum: patient, due to extensive chest involvement the respiration is laboured, and one can even hear the bubbling rales, alae nasi flapping and the patient is struggling for breath. As a rule there is thick-coated tongue, and in spite of the dry lips and tongue there is no thirst. There is loathing to food and in any attempt to feed them there is nausea; with great intolerance to milk. And with their violent cough there is great oppression of the chest and for relief he has to sit up slightly propped up in bed. In these Antimony tart patients there is always a tendency to heart failure with pulse becoming irregular, and heart tends to dilate. Such are the cases seen after the fifth day. For such cases hospitalization is recommended where all the auxiliary methods like oxygen and intravenous fluids etc. will be available.

Carbo vegetabilis: is another drug that has a serious situation like that of Antimonium tart. Both have air hunger but Antimonium tart is more livid and Carbo. veg. is more cyanosed. Both are bathed in sweat but Carbo veg. is extremely cold. The chest has less bubbling but more of consolidated area. Carbo veg. patient responds to oxygen faster and better. As regards the potency — when we are dealing with the acute collapse, dilating heart and heart failure, to obtain a very quick and effective result give high potency and frequent repetition till you get a definite response. There is close resemblance between Kali carb and Carbo vegetabilis.

Kali carb: has violent stabbing pain in the chest with cough. The time of aggravation is mostly in the early hours of the morning say 2 a.m. to 4 a.m. But worse period is 3 a.m. It will be better to prescribe 1m to older patients and higher in the younger patients.

Lycopodium: follows Kali carb. very well. As a rule, Lycopodium is not indicated in the earlier stage of Pneumonia, but often seen after the fourth or fifth day. Normally a carefree and active person develops anxiety and worries that is shown on the forehead with frown. They are domineering and are exacting in their demands on their attendants, and at the same time, want their constant attention. The respiration is always difficult, short, panting and laboured. They complain of tightness of the chest. The sputum is blood-stained, scanty, and difficult to raise. The patients are chilly but dislike stuffy rooms. A definite aggravation between 4 p.m. to 8 p.m. All the complaints like temperature, cough and respiratory distress will increase. Lycopodium respond usually to higher potencies when repeated frequently in pneumonia.

Arsenic alb.: is one of those drugs that are required only in collapse stages of pneumonia. There is intense mental anxiety and restlessness, tossing up in bed till he is physically too tired. It is indicated with the collapse temperature, a running pulse and, possibly, a fibrillating heart. This happens usually early morning between 1 a.m. and 3 a.m. In such cases the Arsenic alb. will start showing reaction unless the remedy is supported by an appropriate complementary remedy like Phosphorus or Sulphur. The response that you will get from Arsenic will be that the patient becomes mentally less anxious, chilliness reduces and warmth appears, the thirst and pulse stabilizes, the temperature begins to rise a little, and at this stage it is time to follow with your complementary remedy — usually Phosphorus.

Sulphur: is an universal remedy and gets indicated at some time or the other or its use as a saviour in difficult situation is observed. Whenever we find that an indicated remedy works positively for some time and progress gets thwarted and we see a picture of some other remedy and, after some time, even that remedy stops working, it is time for Sulphur. It will resolve the condition and stabilize the improvement. At times the temperature comes down but the physical ailments do not reduce keeping the signs at the same level. Sulphur at this point can resolve the issue. In a straight case of Sulphur pneumonia the dirty appearance is characteristic with its red orifices. Weariness with a very low spirit is characteristic. And waves of cold and heat are characteristic. Head and Palms are hot whereas the abdomen is cold, this is due to alteration in the circulation pattern. The cough is very troublesome, cannot raise the mucus with oppressive feeling in the chest. As a rule the left side of the chest is involved. In an acute stage one can go higher, but in the weak or weary stage one should be careful in repeating the remedy.

14. ***The patient gives the history of illness with onset of sore throat and gradual involvement of trachea and larger bronchi, soreness behind the sternum, tightness of the chest, and frequent dry cough and frothy expectoration and elevation of temperature. The physical signs in the chest show patchy consolidation with signs of greater illness. The disease is probably BRONCHO-PNEUMONIA***

The patient looks more ill, with rapid pulse, distressed breathing and mucopurulent sputum rales and ronchi are especially marked at the lung bases. There are reduced breath sounds and tubular breathing. Broncho-pneumonia is more common in winter and spring months. It is often present as a complication of Measles and Whooping cough and other debilitating conditions such as Marasmus or Steatorrhoea.

Antimonium tartaricum: gives sudden alarming symptoms of suffocation and short breath. Accumulation of mucus in the chest, with coarse rattling, must sit up for relief. The pulse is rapid but weak. Dyspnoea is relieved by eructation.

Pulsatilla: Is the next common remedy. In this the patient gives the history of coming out of an attack of measles, dry cough in the evening and at night, must sit up in bed to get relief, expectoration is bland, thick, greenish, bitter. Symptoms are changeable.

Natrum sulph has a slow and gradual onset, hydrogenoid constitution, damp weather always affects: depressed patients, very gloomy, and they do not want to be disturbed and can become quite snappy at times. Very sensitive to noise and get irritated by it. Tongue has grayish green coating, acute pain in the chest while coughing, and needs to hold the side of the chest and sits up, physical restlessness is present. Keeps on changing the position without history of having had a frank cold which has spread down the chest, a very slow advancing progressive pneumonia. The patient gives an impression of having a puffy look, with dusky red coloured face. The patient has marked dyspnoea, with intense tightness of the chest and acute air hunger. They always want open windows and doors and flow of air around them. << in the evening. There is dryness in the mouth with a thick whitish coated tongue but in spite of that there is no thirst. Their most comfortable position is to lie on their back, slightly propped up with hands raised up.

In Kali carb intense dyspnoea although there is great deal of mucus in the chest, it is raised with difficulty. Breathing is whistling and wheezing in character. Often this is a picture after measles.

15. ***The patient complains of sudden paroxysmal attack of difficult breathing with considerable wheezing, but usually without elevation of temperature. The condition is BRONCHIAL ASTHMA.***

Bronchial asthma is characterized by paroxysmal attacks of dyspnoea with short inspiratory effort and prolonged expiration. This is because of narrowing of the trachea, bronchi and bronchioles, specially during expiration. Often there is family history of allergy, e.g. hay fever, migraine, or giant urticaria.

The subject of asthma may be perfectly all right one minute and within minutes may go into a severe attack. The attacks are usually in the early hours of the morning with tightness of chest, cough, gasps for breath, and to breathe needs open windows and fresh air.

There are many interesting features in this disease such as personal history of skin eruptions (urticaria, prurigo, eczema), and these often alternate with the attack of asthma.

We consider Bronchial Asthma as a multi-miasmatic disorder. The expressions of the acute episodes differ from patient to patient depending on the constitutional make up of the individual. It is necessary therefore to recognize these constitutions and their expressions for a successful medical treatment.

Homoeopathy recognizes four constitutional make ups — *The Psoric, The Sycotic, The Pseudo-psoric(Tubercular), and The Syphilitic.*

The Psoric make up is identified through sensitive mental state (Emotional factors), The allergic traits, Suppressed skin disorders/Discharges, and Heredity.

Emotional Factors: Every individual has inherent emotional traits like anger, rage, hate, love, anxiety. The Psycho-Neuro-Endocrine system transmits the emotional attributes to the physical plane. Nostalgic memories of yester years — especially of unpleasant occurrences — can throw a hypersensitive system into spasm. Similarly obsession, under-confidence, sensitive dependent traits, can precipitate Bronchial asthma. Kent's Repertory gives many such emotional symptoms in its chapter on Mind. Similarly, in the chapter of Respiration, two important Rubrics 'Asthmatic' and 'difficult' — are given. They are useful in practice.

Allergic traits: During the development of the human race over millions of years the inherent susceptibility of Man has undergone a tremendous change due to its constant interaction with the environment and, therefore, has become hypersensitive to environment. Allergens like plant pollens, high protein food, sea-food, pesticides, chemicals etc. synthetic clothing, perfumes, industrial waste, fumes, change in weather are responsible for increase of hypersensitivity.

Suppressed skin disorders/discharges: It is observed that, infantile eczema, atopic dermatitis, when treated with topical applications of steroid based ointments or by mercurial preparations travel deep within and are erupted out in the form of Bronchial asthma in later life.

Hereditary : It is one of the strongest factor that transmits these traits during the development of the individual. Qualities, characters and traits derived from both the parents are moulded into patterns which decide your constitution. Subtle changes in the expression of these allergies depend on these constitutions.

In the **Psoric** make up these hypersensitive characters are predominantly seen.

Arsenic alb.: is one of our prime remedy in asthma, whether acute or chronic, with aggravation after midnight and from lying down. Must sit up and bend forward for relief. It is also indicated in cases of asthma which has developed due to bad effects of repercussion of hives.

There is tendency amongst many of us to start the treatment of Bronchial asthma with Arsenic alb. Unless there are clear signs and symptoms of the drug; use of Arsenic should not be resorted to.

Aralia recemosa: the patient is forced to sit up for relief, he feels he would suffocate if he did not. There is a dry wheeze or loud musical whistling respiration. At first the expectoration is scanty and the quantity is more later, and is of saltish taste. There is sensation of foreign body in the throat.

Lobelia inflata: has weak feeling in the pit of the stomach, and is preceded by prickling all over. There is profuse salivation and feeling as of a lump in the stomach.

Bromine: is indicated when the patient feels as if he could not get air enough into his lungs and breathes very deep. It is more so near or at the seashore.

Carbo veg.: is indicated when there is reflex from accumulation of flatus in abdomen. They are greatly relieved by belching out and by hand fanning. They would rush towards the open windows for fresh air.

In the **Sycotic** make up one will find slow and indolent response to any stimulus. Due to constant hostile inputs, the system gets disoriented and tends to lose control which results into appropriate but inefficient aberrant immune response. This causes inefficient metabolic adjustment and result into defective RES (Reticulo Endothelial System) function which, in turn, produces erratic wandering and spasmodic reactions causing cramps, colic and spasm. This also reduces resistance to germs and viruses. The constitution is predominantly hydrogenoid. The aggravations are due to moisture and increased humidity in the atmosphere. The secondary superimposed infections are common which throw the system into spasms and reactive secretions. They cause rattling and humid productive cough. At the mental level, fear complex is enhanced due to dullness in perception and thinking. It causes delusions, hallucinations and illusions. The typical mental states as sadness, indifference, indolence, fear etc., at times are responsible for throwing the system into spasm. These rubrics come handy as 'Ailments from' in preparing the totality.

The typical Sycotic asthma can be identified by running nose, rhinitis, sneezing, with cough and cold. This moves down the chest in due course of time and causes bronchitis, pneumonitis, and wheezing will start which will be aggravated by humidity, sultry hot weather, getting wet in rains and water.

Antimonium Tartaricum: there will be sub-crepitant rales all through the chest, marked wheezing when the child breathes, the cough sounds loose and yet the child cannot raise it. This continues till the child grows drowsy and is bathed in sweat. Gradually cyanosis develops.

Antimonium arsenicosum: another compound of Antimony, is equally useful when the dyspnoea and cough is excessive, with increased mucoid secretions. The anxiety and restlessness is more marked on the face.

Natrum Sulphuricum: is the central remedy for hydrogenoid constitution. It has a marked tendency to develop chest catarrh and any increase in dampness in the weather can cause severe chest congestion with difficulty to breath. Aggravation time is 4 to 5 a.m., cough with thick ropy greenish expectoration.

Stannum metallicum: is another remedy that has great accumulation of mucus in the chest but unless there is great weakness it is rarely indicated. Stannum is a low-spirited individual, and is aggravated by weeping. The dyspnoea is decidedly better after expectoration.

Senega. The remedy of the aged. There is great pressure in the chest as though the lungs were forced back to the spine. Great difficulty in raising the mucus and soreness in the chest wall.

Thuja and **Medorrhinum** are two great remedies of the sycotic or hydrogenoid constitution. Thuja is a chilly patient and the Medorrhinum is hot. Both of these are often used as inter-current or constitutional remedies.

In **Medorrhinum**, asthma is from weakness and or spasm of epiglottis, feels the larynx is stopped, no air can pass. Only relieved by lying on face and protruding tongue. Is better at the seaside when asthma is connected even remotely with gonorrhoeal infection.

In **Thuja** there is short breath from mucus in the trachea, peculiar symptom is sweats only on uncovered parts and has a very offensive odour. Aggravated in damp weather. It often works as chronic of Arsenic alb.

A perfect complement to Arsenic alb. is Kali Bichromicum. The asthma is worse from 3 to 4 a.m. in the morning. The bronchial tubes are filled with thick tenacious mucus and obliges the patient to sit up in bed, bending forward for relief. This asthma often returns every winter or in summer when it is chilly. Lower potency of Kali Bichrom, 4x or 6x is found more useful at times in the treatment of asthma.

The **Pseudo-Psoric** or the **Tubercular** constitution is identified through a very sharp, creative and intelligent personality. But they are physically weak and debilitated. This weakness fails to translate the creative ideas into practice. Frustration develops which at times becomes responsible to develop spasms. They lack energy to draw full breath, cold air aggravates them, when the body is exposed to chill. They seem to revive with the heat of the day and, as the sun descends, they loose the warmth again.

Tuberculinum: is indicated in persons with a history of tuberculosis infection, or a family history of tuberculosis. These subjects take cold very easily everytime he gets a breath of fresh air; but yet craves for fresh air.

Kali carbonicum: has sensation of no air in the chest, and the worse time is 2 to 3 a.m. Kali carb is better sitting upright, slightly forward, bending over the table or knees relieved by rocking. Lying down is impossible, worse by drinking and motion.

Sambucus: has also similar aggravation time and springs out of the bed at that time. Asthma with suffocative attacks. He is well when awake but then sleeps into the attack. Dry heat when asleep, profuse sweat when awake.

Bromium: is having asthma particularly in sailors when they go ashore. They cannot breathe deep enough, sense of constriction and must sit up. Sensation of air passages full of smoke. They are worse from dust. They develop gasping, wheezing, rattling and spasmodic closure of glottis.

The **Syphilitic** constitution is weak and debilitated system that develops over prolonged period of working under stress, reaches to a point of no return and loses the elasticity of alveoli and becomes permeable to improve the ventilation.

Hepar Sulphuris: is one of such anti-syphilitic drug which has anxious wheezing, moist breathing, worse in dry cold air and better in damp cold weather with associated palpitation of the heart.

Mercurius: due to secondary infection to air causing intercellular gap to be filled in reducing the exchange of oxygen : carbon dioxide. This we understand by the name emphysema. Similar destruction takes place in the bronchi and bronchioles which invite infection due to stagnation of air. The right heart gets enlarged and is then followed by hypertrophy. Eventually failure results. These are mostly the non-reversible changes. We classify these destructive non-reversible changes as ***Syphilitic***. The treatment here is more palliative than curative. Because of the advancing pathology, the differentiating symptoms are mostly missing and the picture is mostly the signs of pathology. The conditions like cor pulmonale, emphysema, and status asthmaticus show only pathological picture like breathlessness, restlessness which many drugs have. To arouse the susceptibility within, at times low potency in frequent doses are required and supportive physiological treatment like oxygen and bronchodilators are needed to improve ventilation. We can think of some of these anti-syphilitic drugs like:

Hepar sulphuris: which has anxious wheezing, moist breathing, worse in dry cold air, and better in damp cold weather with associated palpitation of the heart.

Mercurius due to secondary infection in the lungs there is suppuration and bloody thick green expectoration and large quantities of pus. The sweat does not relieve. To bring a quick palliation the lower potency of Mercurius does a excellent job.

Syphillinum: has chronic asthma in summer, and aggravations are at night.

There are some partially proved or short proved remedies like:

Histamine Chloride: This is an allergic remedy of Psoric and Tubercular personality. Often the bronchial symptoms accompany skin symptoms. This can be used where the patient has received large doses of Antihistaminics, during the treatment of Asthma, or for any other ailments.

Berryllium: was an accidental find. Workers working in the Berryllium mines were found to develop lung fibrosis, X-ray showed snowfall appearance, looking like pulmonary sarcoidosis and emphysematous lung. Low potency of this remedy helps to slow down the progress of this disease.

Naphthaline: produces symptoms of hay fever with dyspnoea and sighing respiration. It is useful in emphysema of the aged.

In practice, one will find many patients who are already on some treatment — like bronchodilators, antibiotics, antihistaminics, steroids — will come for homoeopathic advise. Depending on health status of each individual you have to decide whether to allow them to continue their non-homoeopathic treatment if they happen to start the homoeopathic treatment.

Investigations: X-ray may be normal but sputum may contain large number of eosinophils, and peripheral blood film will show more eosinophilia. Simple spirometery or Candle blowing test should be instituted.

16. ***The patient complains of chronic cough, though there is no elevation of temperature, ronchi and rales are heard over the chest. The condition is CHRONIC BRONCHITIS.***

This is an insidious process, normally starting after the age of forty, in persons who are susceptible to respiratory infection. They are usually of sycotic constitution, but in many cases this condition can start after Pneumonia or Influenza. The symptoms start as a cough over a period with mucoid expectoration, sooner or later emphysema develops and breathlessness ensues. In summer it is comparatively better but with the return of damp, foggy and wet weather the symptoms return with acute bronchitis that supervenes. As time goes by the cough and sputum becomes more persistent, and may last the whole year. The patient becomes more breathless with emphysema , marked pulmonary hypertension results and right-sided heart failure may supervene.

Remedies which resemble the pathogenesis are more sycotic in nature, prominently.

Pulsatilla: though chilly prefers outdoors. The discharges are thick, bland and yellowish green. The symptoms always change. Patient is thirstless.

Stannum Iod: has persistent inclination to cough, excited by tickling dry spot in the throat, tracheal and bronchial irritation of the chronic smokers. The cough is loud hollow sounding, ending in an expectoration. Low potency of 3x is more valuable in the chronic condition.

Mercurius: cannot lie on the right side, cough is with yellow muco-purulent expectoration having paroxysms of two, worse at night and from warmth of the bed. Stitching pain in the right lobe of the lung radiating to back.

Antimonium tartaricum: the bronchial tubes are loaded with mucus, the cough is rapid, short and difficult breathing to the point of suffocation. Dyspnoea is relieved by eructation and lying on the right side.

Natrum sulphuricum: is typically a hydrogenoid and sycotic. They are worse in rainy season, in damp weather, and from water in any form. Rattling in the chest in the early hours 3 to 4 a.m., cough is with ropy greenish expectoration.

Senega: is an old man's remedy, rattling in the chest, chest oppressed on ascending, difficulty in raising the mucus, asthenic bronchitis in old people. This is an insidious process normally starting after the age of forty, in persons who are susceptible to respiratory infections, usually of sycotic constitution, but in many cases it may even start after pneumonia or influenza. The symptoms start as cough over a period, with mucoid expectoration, sooner or later emphysema develops, and breathlessness ensues. In summer he is comparatively better but with the return of winter, damp foggy and cold weather, the symptoms reappear with an acute attack of bronchitis that supervenes. As time goes by the cough and sputum becomes more persistent, and may last the whole year, the patient becomes more and more breathless; with the emphysema, marked pulmonary hypertension results and right-sided heart failure may supervene.

Investigations: X-ray chest may show low flat diaphragm and hyperlucent lung fields, there is additional emphysema, Ventilatory indices like ratio of FEV1/FEV is 70% — indicates airway obstruction. Vital capacity is reduced.

Management: To remove the cause as far as possible such as: Air pollution and Smoking, Patient is on a long term treatment with chronic and intercurrent remedies, or constitutional remedies, maintain ambient atmosphere and avoid overheated rooms, damp and foggy places, stuffy clothing, overfeeding, smoking, and too much of alcohol.

17. ***A patient complains of persistent cough, with expectoration, loss of weight and energy, and intermittent pyrexia with occasional frontal headache: night sweats, loss of appetite with fullness of abdomen after a light meal. The condition is PULMONARY TUBERCULOSIS.***

The disease is mainly chronic in nature and its onset is insidious. In fact, in many cases of pulmonary tuberculosis there may be no symptoms and can only be recognized by radiography. Homoeopathy recognizes tuberculosis as a diathesis. For the purpose of treatment we understand that there are premonitory symptoms in 'Pre-tubercular Stage'. To establish a scrofulous state in a body there are some metabolic maladjustments in the digestive sphere described as strumous dyspepsia. The main feature of this dyspepsia is dislike to and difficulty in assimilation of fats, biliousness, heartburn, flatulence, and acid eructation after taking food. If the patient is otherwise well-nourished, he has incapacity to use food containing oil, fat or sugar.

Calcarea carbonica: is related to the pre-tubercular stage of tuberculosis, and mostly suited to disorders of right apical area. Stitching in the chest and sides of the chest while moving about, and while lying on the affected side. The cough is provoked by going in cool room, by chilliness, sensation of feather in the throat. Rattling in the chest. Miller's and Stone cutter's tuberculosis, old suppurating cavities, swelling of cervical and bronchial glands and is a promising remedy as a preventive.

Pulsatilla: three characteristic must be satisfied, Chilly, Worse by warmth, Thirstless. Cough is copious with expectoration. Pressure on the chest and soreness. Shortness of breath, worse lying on the left side, and smothering sensation on lying down, worse in warm and stuffy room. Tickling sensation in the throat causing dry and hacking cough, worse in the evening and night, must sit up in bed to get relief. The expectoration is bland, yellow-greenish, thick purulent, slimy sweet, salty, and bitter as it loosens up.

Iodide of Arsenic: is more important than Arsenic itself. Rapid emaciation and pronounced fever are its chief indications. In the early stage of Tuberculosis, afternoon rise of temperature, profound prostration, rapid, irritable pulse, recurring fever and sweats, emaciation, with nightly drenching sweats are its indications. The lower decimal dilutions are preferred by the older masters (Hughes, Bahr). It is a remedy most closely allied to manifestations of tuberculosis, emaciation and tendency to diarrhoea. Hoarse racking cough, profuse expectoration of a purulent nature. In tuberculous patients there is good appetite but emaciation. It is said that is more useful in lower potency, say 4x, in repeated doses, three times a day.

Stannum iod. and **Kali carb** are two remedies that will be more useful under the circumstances.

Stannum iod: has loud cough with hollow noise ending with expectoration. There is persistent inclination to cough, excited by a tickling dry spot in throat but ever changing its location and, at times at the root of the tongue. The cough starts with a weak sounding accompanied by shortness of breath. The cough soon gathers strength and induces raising of free copious yellow expectoration. Therefore found useful in smoker's cough. Lower potency of 3x is often used.

Kali Carb: has cutting pain in the chest, worse lying on the right side, aggravation in the morning at 3 to 4 a.m., always better in the warm climate, constant taking up of cold that leads to tuberculosis. The cough is dry, paroxysmal, loose viscid mucus or pus which must be swallowed. Easy choking, and food easily gets into the wind-pipe. The expectoration consists of hard white or smoky masses, which fly from throat when coughing. It is a right-sided medicine and the base of the right lung is affected.

Spongia: is the remedy of choice when there is burning and stinging in throat, followed by stitches and dryness. Larynx is painful, dry, constricted, worse on touch, singing or swallowing worsens. Needs to clear the throat constantly. Both glandular system and respiratory system are affected in Spongia. Nocturnal sweats are often the distressing symptoms where Phosphoric acid comes in to help. Whenever the system is exposed to the ravages of severe disease the debility that follows is covered by **Phosphoric acid.**

Tuberculinum bovinum: is a nosode prepared from the tubercular abscess and has an undoubted value in the treatment of incipient tuberculosis. It is mostly indicated in the narrow chested, light complexioned subjects with low recuperative powers, and very susceptible to changes in weather. Very tired person with intense fatigue from any motion. Wants constant changes and aversion to work. When the symptoms are changing, and well selected remedies fail to improve, Tub. is useful. Catches cold with slightest exposure. Tubercular affections of the lung begins from the apex, hard hacking cough, loss of weight and rales all over the chest.

Bacillinum (Burnett): is especially indicated in lungs of old people with chronic catarrhal condition, and weak pulmonary circulation, attacks of suffocation at night with difficult cough. Constant disposition to catch cold. Many forms of non-tubercular diseases are influenced by it.

These two nosodes work well as intercurrent remedies. The most important point is that the patient should need a good protein nourishment, bright sunshine, rest and dry weather. Outdoor exercises are very important.

Investigations: Repeated examination of sputum or laryngeal swab. X-ray chest to observe sub-apical or sub-clavicular patchy shadows. Blood ESR is usually raised. Mantoux test : In active tubercular infection 1 TU, otherwise normally 10 TU is used. Induration less than 5 mm is negative. Erethema and induration should be distinguished.

18. *The patient complains of breathlessness, without any pain or fever. On examination the dullness is found at one or both bases, and signs of fluid are detected. The condition is HYDROTHORAX.*

The commonest cause of this is combination of right and left sided heart failure so that hydrothorax is a part of the cardiac oedema. Malignant disease in the chest is the next possibility — primary bronchial carcinoma, mediastinal tumour or secondary malignant disease arising from a primary focus situated almost anywhere in the body. It can also be part of the general dropsy of sub-acute nephritis when both the pleura are involved. This condition does not have favourable prognosis.

Any effusion left behind by the earlier inflammatory process, tolerably good results will be obtained by Apis. The seniors always vouch by the great drug Sulphur. Here the use of sulphur has been always in very low potency, and frequently daily, and continued for long time. It is claimed that even if the adhesions are formed those will get absorbed and the lung function improves.

19. *Patient complains that for number of years there has been increasing shortness of breath, associated cough and sputum which is often purulent. Local signs are contraction and consolidation in the lungs and clubbing of fingers is usually seen. The condition is FIBROID LUNG.*

Another name to this disorder is Chronic Interstitial Pneumonia. The common cause is chronic pulmonary tuberculosis in middle-aged who have a very high resistance to tubercular bacillus (upper lobes are more involved). There is also a non-tubercular variety where the middle and lower lobes are involved.

Initially there is shortness of breath on exertion but later it occurs even when at rest. There is a progressive diminution of pulmonary function. There is cough with change of position, and therefore marked on waking up.

20. ***The patient complains of breathlessness, which has gradually progressed over the years: there is slight cough with very scanty sputum. The lungs show signs of EMPHYSEMA. There are no local signs but X-ray shows there is considerable degree of fibrosis and, sometimes, nodules. The condition is DIFFUSED FIBROSIS OF THE LUNGS.***

The striking clinical of feature of this disease is shortness of breath and to come to any conclusion X-ray of chest is essential. These changes are as a result of inhalation of dust by the industrial workers (Pneumoconiosis) for a prolonged period . The most hazardous is silicosis (inhalation of Silicon dioxide) although coal-miners and workers working in asbestos and Beryllium mines also develop this condition. In non-industrial causes include sarcoidosis , diffuse systemic sclerosis and after extensive X-ray exposure during the course of treatment.

Carbo veg.: is one of our principal remedy for the condition. Carbo veg. is a product of imperfect oxidation and disintegration is the keynote of the remedy. Its action on the venous capillary circulation causes stagnation of the blood circulation — causing blueness, coldness and ecchymosis of the skin. It develops atonic condition where there is lack of reaction. Laborious breathing, short and quick, worse by walking about,often wants to take deep breath. There is evidence of degenerative diseases of the lungs.

Ammonium carbonicum: has increasing difficulty of breathing and often wakes him up. Every effort to enter a warm room. There is rattling in the chest but very little can be raised. There is hypostatic congestion of the lungs and pulmonary oedema.

Fibrous changes in the tissue are mainly related to tubercular miasm and these degenerative changes are often non-reversible. When we think of the therapeutic measures, remedies will also be considered from the tubercular group.

3 GASTROENTEROLOGY

- Common symptoms of the Gastrointestinal disorders
- Diseases of mouth, tongue and oesophagus
- Acid peptic disease
- Abdominal colic
- Acute Appendicitis
- Acute Bacillary and Amoebic Dysentry
- Cholera
- Acute & Chronic
- Ulcerative Colitis
- Diarrhoea
- Constipation
- Acute & sub-acute
- Hepatitis
- Functional diseases of Liver
- Acute Cholecystitis
- Gall stone Colic
- Pancreatitis

Gastrointestinal diseases are the major causes of ill-health all over the world. Large number of people still suffer from amoebiasis, helminthiasis. Poor hygiene and malnutrition allows the spread of infective organisms. Many infections can be prevented by improved sanitation and education. This is equally true in the developed countries. They are also equally affected because of very refined diets and food additives. In spite of both diagnosis and improved treatment techniques, gastrointestinal diseases comprise of more than 15% of the total load of our practice.

Common symptoms of the Gastrointestinal disorders

Dysphagia : It is difficulty in swallowing. This can be because of a local cause or a part of the generalized disease. Patients often complain of something sticking in their throat or chest during swallowing.

Heartburn is common symptom of acid reflux. This pain can spread to the neck, across the chest and at times it becomes difficult to distinguish it from pain of ischaemic heart disease. This is usually felt when lying down flat at night.

Flatulence is the term used to describe excessive wind in the abdomen. It indicates belching, distension or passage of flatus per rectum.

Hiccups are due to involuntary diaphragmatic contraction with closure of the glottis and are extremely common.

Vomiting is the expulsion of gastric contents through the mouth. This can happen in cases other than gastrointestinal disorders too. Nausea occurs first and is followed by retching where the glottis remains closed and finally the vomiting takes place. Vomiting may occur without nausea. It may also occur in pyloric stenosis.

Diarrhoea is an extremely common condition. A single episode is often because of dietary indiscretion. It is important to know from the patient what he means by the term diarrhoea. It can be either acute or chronic. If it is acute then its infective, causes must be found out.

Steatorrhoea is the passage of pale, bulky stool that contains fat and at times it floats in the lavatory pan and is difficult to flush away.

Constipation is difficult to define. Patients describe differently. Difficult passage of large hard stool, infrequent stools, unsatisfactory stools are termed as constipation by the patient. One must, therefore, find from the patient the exact nature of the stool.

Abdominal pain : Large number of causes can be attributed to this pain. Ascertain the site, intensity, periodicity of the pain. Aggravating and relieving factors should be noted. Any associated symptom including non-gastrointestinal symptoms must be taken into account.

Weight loss is mostly due to anorexia.

Rectal Bleeding should be ascertained accurately, e.g. the site of the bleeding.

1. ***Patient complains of pain associated with redness, swelling and tenderness in the mouth. There is widespread inflammation of the cheek, the tongue and the floor of the mouth or the palate. In severe cases, the patient may complain of offensive breath, enlarged and tender cervical lymph glands and occasionally swollen lips. This condition is STOMATITIS.***

There are several varieties of this *stomatitis: Catarrhal, Aphthous, Ulcerative, Herpetic, Parasitic* or *thrush.* But the homoeopathic therapy remains essentially the same because the symptoms expressed are more or less the same with little change in modalities. These are important for prescribing than the underlying pathology.

Borax: has aphthous inflammation of mucus membrane of the mouth and tongue which bleeds easily, therefore useful in aphthous stomatitis. Ulcers bleed on attempting to eat or to touch, it is a white fungus-like growth and a very important concomitant in diarrhoea. The mouth is hot, mucous membrane around these aphthae bleed easily. Stools are usually green and soft and always contain mucus.

Kali chloricum: produces scorbutic and spongy gums, soft, bleed easily, with foul odour to the breath. The look is very red and like fire, with gray based ulcers. The stomatitis is aphthous and gangrenous.

Mercurius: the whole mouth is moist, one finds a very thick and flabby tongue coated with dirty yellow white coating and offensive odour to the breath. Scorbutic symptoms are present, tongue takes the imprints of teeth. The gums ulcerate and become spongy, recede and easily bleed with excessive salivation.

Nitric Acid: has similar features but does not have the offensive breath like others. The tongue is red and glazed and mapped.The saliva is acrid, the pains in the mouth are pricking in nature, the aphthae are white and pale. Ulcers in the soft palate with sharp splinter like pain. Gums bleed.

Arsenic album: has livid bleeding gums, blisters on the edges of the gum and have ulcerating diarrhoea. Burning is more intense, restlessness compelling motion in spite of weakness. The ulcers are bluish-black with intense burning. Mental irritability is more.

Stomatitis can occur with ill-fitting dentures, or with number of vitamin deficiencies.

2. ***Patient complains of recurring attacks of burning pains beneath the lower part of the sternum, the food appears to stick there on swallowing, distension in the left hypochondrium, and occasionally vomiting of blood, loss of weight. The condition may be CHRONIC OESOPHAGITIS.***

The history will reveal that the whole condition has developed gradually, with burning pain in the lower end of the oesophagus shortly after swallowing solid food or very hot drink or alcoholic spirit. This pain initially may be intermittent but later becomes more continuous, so much so that patient goes on starvation, diet with liquids only and antacids which gives him relief.

He swallows lot of air and saliva which causes distension in the left upper abdomen. In some there is severe spasm at the lower end of oesophagus with regurgitation of alkaline fluid. Initially there may be simply an inflammatory condition but later peptic ulcers may form with minor degree of bleeding, haematemesis, melaena or anaemia. Weight loss is caused because of insufficient food intake.

Arsenic: has characteristic burning pains, these pains are like burning coal of fire and is associated with diarrhoea. The stools are undigested slimy and bloody; the exciting causes are sudden chilling of the stomach with ice water or icecream, alcoholic drinks in excess, bad meat, decayed sausages, rancid fat, overripe fruits etc. Everything that is swallowed seems to lodge in the oesophagus. These burning pains are relieved by external warmth or drinking warm drinks. But are definitely aggravated by cold drinks. The inflammation in the arsenic stomach is aggravated by milk.

Phosphorus: pain in the stomach, better by cold drinks. Regurgitates ingesta by mouthful. Vomiting as soon as soon as the water gets warmed in the stomach. Sharp cutting pains in the abdomen, empty and gall-gone sensation, flatulent colic, worse by hot drinks. It is chronic of Arsenic.

Kali Bichrom.: there is fullness of stomach immediately after meal, particularly after excessive drinking of beer and ale. The vomited matter is sour and is mixed with clear mucus; bitter; and the vomit is renewed after every attempt to eat or drink. It is associated with great deal of distress and burning.

Argentum nitricum: will give history of pain developing immediately after taking food which increases for about an hour followed by vomiting with relief. These patients have strong desire for cold, ice cold sweetened drinks and sweets like icecream.

Carbo vegetabilis: patients develop definite epigastric pains, burning that come on after some time after partaking of food and develop colicky attacks. Anything by way of cold, ice and icecreams will immediately cause great discomfort and distension of stomach with water brash.

Lycopodium: complains of sour stomach and suffering from waterbrash, acute acidity, and recurring attacks of hiccups. They come on more in the late afternoon. In spite of this they are still hungry and their distress increases if they do not partake any food at that time. Cold food aggravates.

We have seen some of the most common remedies in practice. But there are many more worth considering. Important remedies are Pulsatilla, Natrum phos, Natrum carb, Nux vom or Ptelea.

Pulsatilla: is thirstless in almost all complaints, and is aggravated by rich food, fats, pork, pastries, desserts and icecream.

Natrum phos: has complaints with excess of acidity, desires strong tasting things, eggs, fried fish, beer which ameliorates. Has aversion to bread and butter.

Natrum carb: has weak digestion, and it gets aggravated with slightest errors of diet. Gastric pains are better by eating, fats aggravate and drinking cold water after getting overheated causes disturbance.

Nux vomica: has habit of taking stimulants, rich food and late hours of eating, therefore develops irritable digestive system.

Ptelea: there is atonic state of the stomach and is aggravated by lying on the left side. On awaking there is hunger and headache.

3. ***A patient whose temperature is normal complains of a mild epigastric tenderness, nausea, gastric discomfort, headache and depression which comes on suddenly, the condition is ACUTE DYSPEPSIA.***

There is a sudden disturbance of digestion in a previously healthy person, and often occurs after partaking a very heavy meal, excess of alcohol, fats, ice, and many other articles which vary with the idiosyncrasy of an individual. This often is followed by a fit of anger or worry or disappointment.

Acute dyspepsia usually passes off in a couple of days. It may not need any special medication . A very mild emetic like salt water is enough to induce vomiting . A simple milk diet is sufficient for a day or two. A dose of **Nux vomica** or **Pulsatilla**, depending on the type of indiscretion done, would bring the situation under control.

Carbo veg.: is equally important. Patient wakes up in the morning with headache and morning diarrhoea accompanied by great straining. Eructation worse on lying down, fullness of abdomen, burning in stomach. Digestion is slow as it gets putrefied before it gets digested. It is indicated after Nux vom given on symptoms fails to act, although Nux vom has most symptoms of the dyspepsia.

Lycopodium has the immediate distress symptoms. The accumulation of flatulence is more downwards in the lower abdomen as compared to Carbo veg. or Nux vom.

4. ***The patient complains of considerable epigastric pain or discomfort that have come rather suddenly, the condition is probably ACUTE GASTRITIS.***

Majority of these cases are caused by errors of diet, excess of alcohol, and excess of fatty food or rich food. In clinical practice we find from the type of indiscretion that is done in eating and drinking one will seldom need remedies other than Arsenic album.

Arsenic album: is suited to those with excess eating of vegetable diet, melons, strawberries and fruits in general. The stomach is extremely irritable, the least of food and drink causes distress or vomiting or stool or both together. Pain in abdomen causes turning and twisting. The pains are burning in stomach, better by sweet milk. Icecold water distresses the stomach and is vomited out immediately.

Graphites: has sense of pressure in the stomach, sour and foul belching and burning in stomach causing hunger. Better by drinking hot drinks, especially hot milk. Constrictive pain in the stomach with vomiting of food immediately on eating and the stomach is worse by cold.

Hydrastis canadensis: there is more or less constant sore feeling in the stomach, vomits all food but retains milk or water mixed. Sinking and all-gone feeling. Mother tincture and lower potencies act better. (Clifton) Appetite is bad, poor digestion of bread and vegetables and causes belching.

Kali bichromicum: gastric symptoms are relieved after eating but the rheumatic symptoms reappear. The patient feels a sore spot in the stomach, or says there is load of food lying in the stomach. The discharges are thick ropy. Complaints are mostly in the hot weather but at the same time there is liability to catch cold easily. Ill-effects of indulgence in beer and malt liquor.

Nux vomica: has ill-effects of alcohol drugs, spices, stimulants and sexual excesses. Hiccup from overeating, cold or hot drinks. There is nausea in the morning after eating. A sensation of weight in stomach and stomach is very sensitive to pressure. There is ravenous hunger a day before an attack of dyspepsia. Nausea and vomiting with much retching. There is alternate constipation and diarrhoea.

Phosphorus: gastric pains are better by icecream. Water brash, sour taste and sour belching, after every meal, throws up by mouthful in fact when the food gets warm in the stomach. Regurgitation of ingesta in mouthfuls.

There is no evidence that acute gastritis will eventually lead to chronic gastritis or peptic ulceration. Chronic gastritis is seen in pernicious anaemia where there is atrophy of the mucosa which fails to produce the intrinsic factor B_{12}. Three types of chronic gastritis are known Type A (autoimmune,) Type B bacterial gastritis where there is presence of Helicobactor pylori on the surface epithelium and Type C gastritis is recently recognized histologically distinct lesion due to NSAIDS e.g aspirin or pain-killers. Most of these need no treatment but accompanying pernicious anaemia should be treated. Homoeopathic treatment essentially remains the same for both acute and chronic variety.

The remedies listed under acute gastritis are equally useful in the treatment of chronic variety.

5. ***The patient complains of Indigestion. The pain comes on daily with constant relation to food. The pain is relieved by liquid, food and by alkali. There is tenderness and pain on pressure. The condition is probably an ULCER.***

Simple or peptic ulcer is fairly common. The ulcers probably arise by peptic digestion of the stomach mucosa which is injured by local trauma, by toxins swallowed from mouth. The most common are the frequent ingestion of painkillers and steroids. They tend to heal readily unless there is persistent and static gastric hyperacidity.

Usually the complaint passes off by observing a fast or drinking cold milk, or some alkaline mixture. A common prescription for such a condition arising from excess of lactic acid, resulting from too much sugar, sour vomiting and sour eructations.

Natrum phosphoricum: useful in lower potency 4x or 6x. Canine hunger, all-gone sensation, desires strong tasting things, eggs, fried fish, and beer that relieves. Aversion to bread.

Argentum nitricum: there is gnawing ulcerative pain, burning constrictive pain in the stomach. The pains are radiating. Ineffectual attempt at eructation and belching accompanies most of the gastric complaints. Great flatulence and painful swelling in the pit of the stomach. Irresistable desire for sugar and sweets.

Ornithogalum umbellatum: has increased pains while the food passes the pyloric outlet. And there is frequent passing of offensive flatus. There is vomiting of coffee ground coloured matter suggesting haemorrhage.

Psorinum: there is sour, rancid, tasting and smelling like rotten eggs belching but always hungry must have something to eat at night, water brash when lying down.

Phosphorus: pain in the stomach is better by drinking cold water, throws up food by mouthful and the water is thrown up as soon as it gets warm in the stomach. There is acid dyspepsia with bloated abdomen, faint feeling in the epigastrium, not better by eating. Nausea at the thought of food. There is tobacco dyspepsia.

6. ***Patient complains of severe boring pain produced by intake of food and relieved by vomiting. The vomit at times contains streaks of blood. The condition is ACUTE PEPTIC ULCER. Ulcers may be small and multiple.***

Pain is of distending type or boring, aggravated by food; it is relieved by vomiting; the vomitus may contain excess of hydrochloric acid, there may be painless haematemesis, though the appetite is normal, the patient eats less because of the pain he experiences. The choice of remedy is once again:

Natrum phos : and some times Acid sulph. Patient has heartburn, sour eructation, and this often happens after excessive alcohol. Has aversion to coffee and desire for fresh food. There is coldness in the stomach that is relieved by warmth. Patient must be advised to rest in bed. In case of perforation immediate laparotomy must be arranged. If there is intractable vomiting, iced citrated milk is started as early as possible.

Dysentery bacillus (Dys. Co.): Pain in the stomach is worse from eating. Chronic indigestion, Eructation and heartburn, at times nausea in the morning on waking, which is relieved by eating. Heartburns at times sometime after food. Mental strain reacts on the stomach. Pain as a rule is better by lying down. Often very useful in duodenal ulcers.

Hydrastis can: Weak digestion, gastroduodenal catarrh, cutting colicky pains, better after passing flatus, griping pain with the stool. Sore feeling in the stomach, more or less constant. Atonic dyspepsia belching of sour fluid. Vomits all that is eaten, except milk. This causes marasmus.

Phosphorus (See under ulcers).

7. ***Usually a middle-aged person, or an elderly man, or young/middle-aged woman who is enfeebled by illness and anxiety complaining of indigestion or at regular intervals after food, which is relieved after taking light food, by vomiting or by antacids. The condition is CHRONIC GASTRIC ULCER.***

Chronic indigestion with epigastric pains frequently after food that comes on half an hour to two hours after. Pains radiate to left upper abdomen or back, they are located in definite area depending on the site of ulcers in the stomach. The pains are described as aching and gnawing. Patient takes food with caution, usually light liquid diet. Antacids usually relieve the pains.

Nux vomica: is the remedy that strikes first. It is preeminently the remedy for many of the conditions incident to modern life. His indoor life, mental work, lack of exercise and frequent use of stimulants, coffee and alcohol in excess, is the main cause. In order to calm down, the nerves resort to sedatives. This reflects on his digestion and ultimately ends into gastric ulcer.

Antimonium crudum: is yet another remedy that has been found useful. Although has loss of appetite there is a strong desire for pickles and acids. Eructation tastes of food ingested, associated with heartburn and nausea. Bread, pastry, acids, sour wine cause these epigastric pains. Thickly white -coated tongue is the true guiding symptom.

Graphites: is another important remedy. There is nausea and vomiting after each meal, pressure in the stomach, burning that causes hunger, recurrent gastralgia pain temporarily relieved after vomiting, hot drinks and lying down.

Argentum nitricum : has flatulent dyspepsia, belching after every meal, irresistible desire for sugars, and sweets.

Kali Bichromicum : gastric symptoms are relieved after eating but rheumatic symptoms reappear. Sensation of sore spot in the stomach with a load nausea and vomiting after beer.

Lycopodium: has great weakness of the digestion, with much bloating. Hunger but quick satiety. Gnawing pains are better by drinking warm drinks.

Phosphorus: has pain in the stomach, worse by eating, but better by cold drinks; sour taste and sour belching after every meal, and throws up food by mouthful. Vomiting as soon as the water gets warm in the stomach, vomiting is sour bile blood and coffee ground. There is vomiting after post-operative anaesthetic effect of chloroform.

Sepia: acid dyspepsia with bloated abdomen, from over-lifting and by tobacco, boiled milk disagrees. Burning in the pit of the stomach, and nausea in the morning before eating.

8. ***The patient is healthy looking, active and has been complaining about frequent attacks of acidity for many years, after overwork, worries or taking indigestible foods: develops pain 3-4 hours after meals or in the night, that is relieved by eating food or antacids. The condition is*** **CHRONIC DUODENAL ULCER.**

The symptoms of this condition begins early in life and comes in the form of attacks after dietetic irregularity, subsequently the attacks last for longer period and they come on sooner than previous attacks. The epigastric pains are some times intense, usually nagging or gnawing. This is usually almost quickly relieved after eating. The pains may migrate to the back or become more constant if the ulcer burrows the head of the pancreas. X-ray or endoscopy clinches the diagnosis.

As the symptoms suggest the first remedy that strikes is:

Nux Vomica: The circumstances and the situation points to this remedy. Nux vomica suits those who indulge in excess of alcohol, indigestible food, irregular habits, lack of sleep, loves fatty food and tolerates them very well, and lot of coffee drinking, there is constipation with frequent ineffectual urging, incomplete and unsatisfactory stools.

Pulsatilla: has an aversion to fatty food, warm food and drink. Eructation taste of food long remaining in the stomach, after iced drinks, fruits and pastries. There is often bitter taste in the mouth. Like Nux vom there is pain in abdomen an hour after eating.

Graphites: has nausea and vomiting after each meal. Sweets nauseate and aversion to meat and hot drinks disagree. Constrictive pain in the stomach, recurrent gastralgia. Stomach pain is temporarily relieved by eating. Dyspepsia due to farinaceous and fermentable foods, cabbages, beans.

Lycopodium: Has desire for sweet things, food tastes sour, great bulimia, eating, just a little flatulence. Always likes to take hot food. Burning eructation rises up to throat and remains for long.

Apart from the remedial therapy more important is the auxillary management of such patients. Patient must be given mental and physical rest, nourishing food that does not cause any digestive errors. Overwork, worry or stress should be avoided. Initially the attack may last for a few days but these efforts reduce the superacidity of the gastric juice, gradually returning to normal work in nearly three to four months.

9. ***The patient complains of constant abdominal pain which aggravates especially after exercise, associated nausea or vomiting with some elevation of temperature with rapid pulse: there is rigidity and tenderness in the right iliac fossa region, the disease is ACUTE APPENDICITIS.***

In clinical practice two types of this conditions are seen. One is catarrhal inflammation of the vermiform appendix, and the second is virulent form with ulceration, gangrene and local or diffuse peritonitis.The symptoms are characteristic; point to appendix pain, vomiting, tenderness, local rigidity, quickened pulse and leucocytosis. Initially the pain is generalized over the abdomen, epigastrium and then settles in the right iliac fossa. MacBurney's point is tender on pressure.

Patient complains of violent colic, that comes and disappears suddenly. The tenderness of the abdomen is worse by least jar. The pain is throbbing, localized in the ileo-caecal region and cannot bear slightest touch. Even the bed-clothes are very sensitive. Face is red with dilated pupils. These symptoms point to Belladonna.

Belladonna: is more useful at the early inflammatory stage much before the suppuration has set in that means when there is generalized pain in the abdomen but when the pains become localized there are more chances of the suppuration developing. Belladonna may hasten this suppuration and can burst the inflammed appendix causing peritonitis. Under the circumstances use Plumbum met.

Plumbum met: There is violent colic and the patient assumes the strangest postures for relief. The pains radiate to all parts of the body. Violent colic cause the abdominal muscles to retract till navel seems to press against the spine.

Magnesia phos: where we find spasmodic cramping of stomach nipping, gripping, and pinching with belching that does not relieve. Flatulent colic that forces the patient to bend and better by warmth and rubbing. Use 12x, or 1M .

In chronic appendicitis, there is pain starting from right iliac fossa or radiating from umbilicus or epigastrium to this region. Usually after food and aggravated by overexertion. Prolonged retention of barium in X-ray will confirm the diagnosis. Filling defect will be present. With any malignant disease, tuberculosis, stricture of lumen with formation of mucocoele of the appendix.

One remedy that I have found very useful is Iris tenax. I have used this in number of cases where there is dry mouth, deathly sensation at a point in the stomach and pain in the ileo-coecal region. Repeated low potency doses help. This needs to be differentiated from acute amoebic colitis.

10. ***Patient is complaining of sudden and severe pain in abdomen, doubling up with restlessness, or rolling about in cold sweat, often there is vomiting, the face is pale and anxious, feeble, rapid pulse, without any temperature, no physical signs in abdomen but may be relieved by pressure. The condition is INTESTINAL COLIC.***

The intestinal colic is due to distension and spasm of the bowel. The spasm of the small intestine is characteristically twisting and is paroxysmal in nature and refers to epigastrium or umbilicus. The colic of the colon is referred to hypogastrium. The palpating hand can appreciate the hardening of the bowel. Relief from pressure distinguishes it from peritonitis. At times it is accompanied by diarrhoea.

Plumbum met: Excessive colic that spreads all over abdominal wall, feeling of abdominal wall being retracted, severe constipation, stools hard and lumpy. Plumbum is very useful in intestinal obstruction, intussusception and hernia.

Carbo. vegetabilis: one will find gaseous distension with wind colic belching that relieves.

Colocynthis: has agonizing cutting pain in abdomen, intestines feel bruised, the colics appear after anger, least food or drink brings on dysenteric stool and the colic are better by bending double.

Mercurius: has stabbing pain in the abdomen with flatulent distension, dysenteric stools with or without blood.

Chamomilla: Abdomen distended, spells of flatulent colic, after anger. Cutting wind colic, aggravated at night, better by warm application.

11. ***The patient who is a professional/regular traveller complains, more or less, sudden diarrhoea with mucus and sometimes blood in the stools; constitutional symptoms with pyrexia, headache and abdominal pain, followed by dehydration. The condition is ACUTE BACILLARY DYSENTERY.***

Bacillary dysentery is common in tropical and subtropical climates. After an incubation period of 1-7 days there is a sudden onset of fairly high fever, nausea, vomiting and headache followed by colicky abdominal pain, tenesmus and frequent passage of small stools. As the toxaemia increases the face becomes flushed, pulse becomes rapid and tongue gets coated. The general picture of dehydration becomes evident with sunken eyes, pinched features, restlessness, and, in infants, depressed fontanelles. Soon the foecal character of the stool is lost and it becomes gelatinous mucus mixed with bright red blood.

Before we decide of its various remedies we need to understand the cause and occurrence: Type of stool; concomitants, before, during, and after the stool; and modalities. A quick reference to the repertory will help to come to a conclusion of the remedy in every case.

In clinical practice the most important and often indicated remedies in acute condition are Nux Vom., Mercurius, Merc corrosive, Trombidium, Arsenic alb, Aloe, Nitric acid.

Nux vom: there is frequent and scanty stool, with marked urging. Stool relieves the pain for some time to return again after some time.

Mercurius: has a never-get-done feeling, bloody slimy stools with much straining.

Merc cor: is more violent than Merc sol. Slime and wet tongue with excessive thirst is characteristic. Chilliness is followed by stool. There is more blood than in Merc sol.

Trombidium: is worse by food and drink. Urgent loose stool after rising from bed.

Arsenic: there is putrid, involuntary stools, frequent thirst for small quantity but the most important is restlessness and anxiety.

Aloe: there is fullness of abdomen, heavy, hot and bloated. Sense of insecurity in the rectum. A lot of mucus that passes after the stool with pain in the rectum.

Nitric acid: there is great straining but very little stool passes. Violent and cutting pain in the rectum that remains long after the stool. But passes profuse and bright blood.

12. ***The patient is a child, developing sudden, at first yellow and offensive stool, then greenish and slimy and often mixed with undigested food. The condition is ACUTE CATARRHAL INFANTILE DIARRHOEA.***

13. ***The patient is a child, develops greenish, stools slimy, containing mucus, and streaks of blood. There is slight fever in the beginning with abdominal distension in the colonic area. But the colour, and consistency of the stool changes with type of infection. The condition is ENTEROCOLITIS OR INFLAMMATORY INFANTILE DIARRHOEA.***

14. ***The patient is a child, the stools are watery, foul smelling, green in colour, containing mucus, which starts suddenly but insidiously. There may be vomiting followed by dehydration, elevated temperature, prostration and collapse. The condition is EPIDEMIC DIARRHOEA.***

The above three conditions are fairly common in children during their first one year of life, mostly because of bad hygiene, contaminated water and summer warmth. Some of the infections are because of organisms like *shigella, flexener* and *sonne* and *b. coli* or *e. coli staphylococci.* In many epidemics no infection can be detected — then it is treated as viral infection.

By whatever name the conditions are labeled the homoeopathic remedies do not differ very much because of the indications of these remedies are on the basis of presenting signs and symptoms, which remain often very same. Only what is important is the modalities, circumstances of its appearance and the concomitants.

Aconite: is indicated when there is sudden, green, watery, frequent stools caused due to chill or fright; or suppressed perspiration,

Bryonia: is indicated when there is unquenchable thirst, and diarrhoea is from hot weather.

Dulcamara: when the weather changes to cool or exposure to cold weather, colic before the stool.

Croton tig.: watery stool comes out like shot while nursing or immediately after. Chamomilla has watery greenish stools smelling like rotten eggs, very irritable, uncivil and snappy child.

Gambogia: Pain in the stomach after food, tenasmus after stool with burning in anus, sudden forcible ejection of bilious stool, mostly in elderlys and in hot weather.

Veratrum alb: diarrhoea is with violent vomiting, cold sweat on the forehead with the slightest activity.

Podophyllum: has painless, profuse stools, offensive, gushing and causes a quick dehydration. Desires much water to drink but not to eat any food. This diarrhoea is worse in the morning and there is a normal natural stool in the evening usually during teething in babies.

Bacillus Gaertner (Bach): is a bowel nosode, very useful in babies who have this coeliac disorder after they have been put on the top feed. In slightly older children they cannot digest fatty food, although they desire puddings, milk, sweets, eggs. Vomit after sweets, their diarrhoea is fetid, every fifteen days mixed stool with mucus and blood.

15. ***The patient complains of sudden diarrhoea, attended with severe collapse, abdominal cramps, and 'rice water stools' — the condition is probably CHOLERA.***

Often known as Asiatic cholera, a condition caused by organism Cholera vibrio. It begins with urgent vomiting, purging and colourless evacuations.

Cuprum arsenicosum: is the most valuable remedy having rumbling and sharp cutting pains in the abdomen followed by cold clammy sweat of intermittent character. There are cramps in the calves. Repeated lower potencies help.

Veratrum album: is another remedy that very much simulates Cholera. Sinking and empty feeling in the abdomen, Diarrhoea is very painful, watery, copious and forcibly evacuated followed by great prostration. Vomiting accompanies the purging. Intermittent cold clammy sweat.

Camphor is the third of Hahnemann's cholera remedy. Everything is vomited, the tongue is blue and cold, and breath is cold too; cold sensation in the stomach. In cold stage wants to uncover and in hot phase wants to remain warm.

Arsenic alb : Effect of food poisoning, caused by bad meat, vegetables, water, melons and watery fruits. Dyspepsia from acidic, icecream , vinegar. Burning pain in the stomach.

16. (a) ***Patient complains of sudden onset of diarrhoea, with pain in abdomen occurring in paroxysms, with dark, offensive stools, a mixture of blood and mucus; complains of tenderness over the ascending colon. Pyrexia of 101° to 103°F. The condition is ACUTE ULCERATIVE COLITIS.***

(b) ***The patient complains of augmented form of above conditions, having developed insidiously; from (i) simple diarrhoea, comprising of watery stools mixed with bright blood, mucus and faeces. (ii) lower abdomenal flatulence, (iii) rectal discomfort (iv) Considerable number of stools with dehydration, (v) marked weight loss, and anaemia. This condition is CHRONIC ULCERATIVE COLITIS.***

In the absence of any infective organism having been detected,this condition is regarded as purely psychogenic in origin. Stress, unresolved conflicts, business worries, financial burdens and impositions of sudden responsibilities. Strong Psoric and Syphilitic traits (Tubercular) inherent in the individual bring forth this condition.

Intermissions are common, apparent recovery is followed by relapses and a long term treatment is therefore necessary.

Ignatia: Since the emotional element is uppermost in Ignatia, relationship of this physical irritation first needs to be established. To resolve this emotional state infrequent doses of high potency will be required as intercurrent medication.

Natrum mur: is chronic of Ignatia. Ill-effects of grief, fright and anger aggravations by consolation are the characteristic features. Cutting pain in abdomen, and the abdominal ring, burning and stitching pain in the rectum after a copious diarrhoea.

Staphysagria: is a nervous personality with marked irritability. This irritability is reflected in temper as well as in the function of the digestion. The peristalsis is aggravated with the emotional outburst.

Aurum met: has feeling of self-condemnation and utter worthlessness, profound despondency that affects the digestion.

Nux vom: If one studies the pathogenesis of Nux Vom, one sees a clear picture of this condition. I have found it extremely useful in the treatment of ulcerative colitis, both in acute as well as chronic state when apparently indicated remedies fail to evoke response.

Lycopodium: is another remedy that has a very close resemblance to the condition.

Mercurius solubilis or corrosive: both have a very close relationship with the pathology of ulcerative colitis.

Bacillus sycoccus (Paterson): a bowel nosode has a very close resemblance to the pathogenesis of ulcerative colitis. Person of tubercular constitution, a nervous anxiety, tense and tearful. There is chronic irritation of the alimentary tract, heartburn and hyperacidity, there is urgent desire to stool on waking up in the morning. Stools are loose and offensive.

Cynodon dactylon: one of the indigenous remedy which was added to our remedy list recently. It has griping pains and dysenteric symptoms aggravated by anger and anxiety. It works better either with Mercurius or Nux vom.

Apart from the treatment through the remedies, a lot of counselling and appropriate diet regimen is required.

Correction of dehydration and electrolyte losses through intravenous fluids may often be required which may not be possible at home and need admission to the hospital. Similarly, correction of anaemia by blood transfusion to maintain the haemoglobin level should be done. Initially water by mouth but later high roughage diet may be suggested.

17. ***The patient complains of afebrile diarrhoea, with several voluminous foetid stools daily containing brownish mucus and red blood. Tenesmus is present. The condition is probably ACUTE AMOEBIC DYSENTERY.***

This protozoal amoebic dysentery is common in tropical areas where there is faulty and contaminated water supply, and infected vegetables that are partaken. A stool examination can confirm the diagnosis. The infection is largely affecting the large intestines and the complications can produce intestinal haemorrhage, perforation with peritonitis, retrocoloic abscesses and post-dysenteric adhesions, amoebic liver.

In clinical practice we come across the pathogenesis of three remedies very close to the symptomatology of amoebic dysentery. Nux vomica, Merc sol, Merc cor are closely related.

Nux vomica: has ineffectual desire for stool, unsatisfactory feeling, temporarily feeling better after passage of stool.

Merc sol.: has never-get-done well feeling with passage of large quantity of mucus and less blood. The tongue is moist and flabby, taking the imprint of the teeth, thirst although the tongue is moist. But in Merc cor there is plenty of blood and mucus with increased pain. The bouts of pain come intermittently.

Low residue diet is advised. Weak tea, curds and buttermilk in large quantity is better. Must avoid high proteins, deep fried food, meat and oily fish. Similarly green leafy vegetables should be avoided. It is advisable to wash the pre-cooking vegetables in potassium chloride solution to disinfect the vegetable.

Trombidium: is another remedy that comes handy. There is severe pain in abdomen before and after the stool with griping pain in the hypochondrium.

Nitric acid: has violent cutting pain after the stool, lasting for hours.

Gambogia: has a diarrhoea very similar to Cróton tig. Yellow coloured stool is expelled all at once after considerable urging followed by a feeling of great relief, and it is preceded by excessive cutting around the navel. Burning in anus after stool.

18. ***The patient complains of delay in the passage of contents of the intestine, causing hard, dry faeces. This condition is CONSTIPATION.***

Patients attribute this condition by various ways. Little quantity of stool, irregular stool, painful evacuation, has to strain a lot to evacuate, etc. Symptoms that accompany or result from constipation are very familiar; headache, languor and depression, furred coated tongue, dyspepsia, urticarial eruptions. Habitual constipation may give rise to haemorrhoids. Often the main cause of constipation is errors of diet. Too bland, too dry, too rough and irritating food or too little or poor food is responsible for this. Similarly, sedentary habits, lack of exercise, depression or anxiety contribute to this condition.

Arsenic album: its pathogenesis corresponds to several severe types of diseases that make its homoeopathic application constant and certain — that burning pain in abdomen like coal fire, better by sweet milk, an unconquerable chronic constipation — mostly from inaction or paresis with loss of appetite. Faeces at times protrude and recede or involuntary after fright.

Plumbum: has habitual obstinate constipation, paresis of intestines. There is urging and terrible constriction and spasm of the anus, violent colic with the sensation of abdominal wall being pulled back towards the spine.

Alumina: has inactivity of the rectum and has great straining at stool — even to pass a very soft stool. This may develop because of constant use of aluminium utensils.

Conium: Inability to strain at stools usually due to senile state. A very unusual symptom is that he sweats profusely in sleep or on closing the eyes. Straining at stool causes uterine prolapse.

Silicea: has stool of hard lumps, straining till abdominal wall becomes sore. Shy stool returns back after showing.

Sanicula: has no desire till a large accumulation is collected, stool is so hard that it is impossible to evacuate. Head sweats profusely at night.

Magnesium mur: is worse from salt and at seaside, stool crumble at the anus.

Nux vomica: one will find unsatisfactory stools with ineffectual desire to pass stool. Mostly in literary type who are engaged in studies and exerting of mind, with sedentary habits without any outdoor exercises.

Bryonia: there is no desire. Stool is too thick and large, charred black, and after the stool long continued burning in rectum.

Natrum mur: has obstinate retention of stool irregular hard and dry. Often during menstrual period. Very irritable, weepy and hates fuss. Craves salt.

Graphites: has a large stool, hard knotty, mixed with tough slimy mucus. There is relief from eating hot foods and drinks.

Opium: has obstinate constipation, no desire to go to stools, hard round blackballs, faeces protrude and recede.

19. ***Patient complains of pain in the gall bladder area. This pain is paroxysmal, or dull and continuous, and it radiates to the right shoulder. There is tenderness over the gall bladder, vomiting and fever. The condition is ACUTE CHOLECYSTITIS.***

Berberis vulgaris: affects the liver markedly, promotes the flow of bile, therefore it is useful remedy for fleshy people with good livers but having poor endurance. Sticking pain in the region of the liver shooting up to the right shoulder, worse by pressure. Constipation with gall stone colic with severe pain and yellow complexion. There is heartburn and nausea before breakfast and is better after breakfast.

Carduus mar: has its action centered round the liver and portal system causing soreness and pain, jaundice: There is general oedema, stitches in the liver, worse lying on the left side.

Chionanthus vir: patient is better lying on abdomen there is heat but aversion to uncover, very bitter eructation, constant nausea and retching with desire for stools.

Natrum sulph: is an important remedy for gall stone colic. There is a sensation of lump below the liver and crawling in the liver. Cannot take deep breath without pain. Worse in damp weather. Nux vom is oversensitive and touchy. Liver is swollen, indurated sensitive to pressure and stinging. Cannot bear tight clothing.

China: has pain in the hepatic region, worse from touch and least pressure. There is periodic recurrences with yellow skin and conjunctiva, constipation with dark green scybala.

Chelidonium: has pain travelling backwards or fixed at the angle of right scapula has enlarged liver, jaundice is because hepatic and gall bladder obstruction.

Yingling reports that when it is absolutely impossible to take symptoms during the attack, **Cholesterinum** in low potency does a better job.

20. ***Patient is middle-aged or elderly — is seized suddenly with violent upper abdominal pain, at times radiating to the lumbar region: Vomiting is severe, the abdomen is distended, the bowels are constipated and severe shock with vasomotor collapse develops. The condition is likely to be an ACUTE PANCREATITIS.***

Our literature recommends many remedies for the pains of pancreatic colic. and all of them are equally good when they match the symptoms. But what is found most useful in our daily practice is that great anti-spasmodic.

Belladonna: there is extreme sensitiveness, specially to jarring. The face is red and hot. Extreme irritability of the nerve centers. Excitability.

Calcarea carb: has colic around the navel with darting pain from right to left. Profuse sweat about the head when rest of the body is warm. Sensation of cold damp stockings in the legs. Desire for eggs and boiled eggs. Chronic of Belladonna.

Berberis: is an excellent remedy for both renal and biliary calculi. There is sudden stabbing like pain in the liver, sits bent over pain on the painful side for relief, sticking pain under border of false rib — Haemorrhagic Pancreatitis.

21. ***Repeated attacks of above condition causes the fibrosis of the organ followed by mild attack of jaundice, the condition is CHRONIC PANCREATITIS.***

The pain is very sudden in onset, persistent and severe in the midline, or to the left or right of the upper abdomen, the pain the lumbar area is less in intensity, severe and repeated vomiting with constipation. Vasomotor collapse with thin thready pulse, low blood pressure and sweating. Serum amylase is raised and glycosuria and hyperglycaemia may be found.

Phosphorus: is one of the few remedies that are known to act on pancreas. The characteristic symptoms of phosphorus, desire for cold water, characteristic fears, and haemorrhages.

Iodine: has affinity for glands, it cannot stand warmth, pain in the pit of the stomach top navel and back. Profound debility and great emaciation.

Iris versicolour: causes acute affections of the pancreas, inflammation or salivation, Bilious acrid stools burn like fire.

22. ***Patient feels unwell with nausea, vomiting and diarrhoea, anorexia, headache malaise and distaste for cigarettes. There is mild fever, and a slight upper abdominal discomfort with tender liver. The condition is HEPATITIS.***

This is the prodromal or pre-icteric phase of the disease which lasts up to 2 weeks. The viraemia causes the patient feel unwell with nausea, vomiting, diarrhoea, anorexia, headache and malaise. After 1 or 2 weeks the patient becomes icteric, and may show signs of improvement. The appetite returns and the patient feels better. As the jaundice deepens the urine becomes dark, the stools turn pale due to intrahepatic cholestasis. The liver is moderately enlarged and spleen is palpable There may be transient rash. Thereafter the jaundice reduces and, in majority of cases, the illness is over in 3-6 weeks time, there is rarely a relapse. But if relapse appears, then jaundice returns. The prognosis is very good and most cases completely recover. Patients may complain of debility for several months following resolution of the symptoms and biochemical parameters. This is Hepatitis A and is commonest of viral hepatitis. Its spread is through faecal-oral route and arises from ingestion of clams, shellfish or water. Over-crowding and poor sanitation is another important cause.

Hepatitis B virus spreads through intravenous route. Transfusion of infected blood, contaminated needles, used by drug addicts, tattooist, or accupunturist. or by sexual contacts particularly in male homosexuals. From mother to child during parturition or soon after birth is the most important means. Clinical features are the same as those found under Hepatits A infection. Majority of cases recover completely. Prevention is by avoiding the risk factors.

Hepatitis C is due to an RNA virus (HCV). Seen in intravenous drug abusers and male homosexuals. There are more extra hepatitis manifestations including arthritis, agranulocytosis, and aplastic anaemia and diffuse neurological problems. Progression to chronic liver disease.

Chelidonium: is one of our greatest liver remedy. It acts on portal system, right side of the abdomen and right lower lung. It covers many of the direct reflex symptoms of the diseased condition of liver. It manifests the congestion inflammation, fullness and enlargement in semi-chronic and acute cases. The keynote of the remedy is tearing, shooting stitching pains from the liver region travelling to the back below the right shoulder blade. Hot drink and hot milk relieves.

Bryonia: inflammation of the liver — the right lobe of the liver is mostly affected and feels like a load in the hypochondrium. Every slightest movement hurts, with burning and stitching pains and nausea.

Podophyllum: there is congestion and enlargement of the liver with great irritability of the liver, slight rubbing of the liver helps, the discomfort is aggravated by the slightest thought or smell of food.

Carduus mar.: has feeling of engorged liver, pressure feeling worse by lying on the left side, left liver is full and engorged and sensitive. Concomitant symptoms here are haemoptysis due to congestion of the liver and lungs.

Ptelea trifoliata: has aching in the liver aggravated by lying on the left side, voracious or poor appetite. Develops a repugnance to animal food, rich puddings, of which he is very fond of, butter and fats aggravate his hepatic symptoms.

Lycopodium: has sore pain in the right hypochondrium which is aggravated by touch. Intense flatulence by 4 p.m. as if everything that he takes turns into gas or wind, better by warm drinks.

Phosphorus: has hyperaemia and enlargement of the liver. Craves cold food and drink, icecream and wine, has bad effects of excessive intake of salt. As soon as the cold water becomes hot in the stomach he vomits. Phosphorus is useful when there is suppuration in the hepatitis, hectic fever, night sweats and marked soreness over the liver.

Arsenic: which is acute of Phosphorus has burning thirst and drinks bit by bit, but warm water. This burning of arsenic is better by warm application. There is typical Arsenic anxiety and restlessness.

Nux vomica has constrictive pains in the region of the liver, the liver is swollen, indurated, and sensitive with pressure. Aversion to meat, tobacco and coffee, ale etc., The patent is chilly and irritable. Other remedies and their prescribing indications are the same as mentioned.

Myrica cerifera. It has marked action on the liver and heart, distinctive features are aching pain in the liver, fullness, dull heavy headache, worse in the morning, weakness with ash-coloured stools, slow pulse and pain under the scapula. Jaundice of all degrees. Low potency found to be working better.

Cornus circinata has caused liver derangement, with aching eyeballs, disturbed sleep, Weakness in the morning, pain in the pit of the stomach, with distended abdomen. Dark foul stools, burning in anus, vesicular eruption on the face.

23. ***Patient complains of sudden development of malaise, anorexia, and fever, slightly enlarged liver and yellow tinged conjunctiva. Occasionally there may be pale stools, and dark urine. The condition is ACUTE LIVER DISEASE.***

Acute parenchymal liver damage can be caused by many agents and the extent of damage can be variable.

Hepatitis A is commonest type of viral hepatitis. Is often in epidemics worldwide. Mostly in autumn and affects young children and adults. Shell fish and clams are the common items which infect.

The prodromal phase lasts up to two weeks, and this viraemia causes the patient to feel unwell with nausea, vomiting and diarrhoea, anorexia, headache and distaste for cigarettes. There is an upper abdominal discomfort, and, at times, mild fever. The liver is tender but not enlarged initially. Icterus develops one to two weeks after, at times. All these symptoms may improve, appetite returns and patient feels better. Occasionally there is tender lymphadenopathy and rash in some cases. Liver biochemistry may be performed. Most patients make a complete recovery.

Homoeopathy offers a clear line of treatment irrespective of the liver pathology. The remedies enumerated above under hepatitis cover the pathogenesis of almost every Hepatic disorder. It must be remembered that the final selection of the remedy will be based on the totality of the case. The list above enumerates the various remedies which have close resemblance to the liver pathology.

24. ***Middle-aged person gives a history of chronic dyspepsia, haematemesis, recurrent ascites, and a small hard liver, and an enlarged spleen, and presents with a congested facies. The condition is CIRRHOSIS of the liver.***

Cirrhosis results from the necrosis of liver cells followed by fibrosis, and nodule formation. This causes change in the architecture of the liver which interferes with the blood flow and the function. This change produces clinical features of portal hypertension and impaired liver cell function.

Carduus marianus: the action of this remedy is centered in the liver and portal system. Causing soreness, pain and jaundice. The remedy is suited for those who had ill treated their liver with alcohol, beer in particular. The liver is engorged, swollen laterally and painful to pressure. Cirrhosis with general oedema, left lobe very sensitive, Stitches in the liver worse lying on the left side. The liver disorder causes lung disorder.

China officinalis: there is fermentation in the bowel, frothy and sour-smelling diarrhoea, yellow watery, with much flatus but painless, stools are frequent at night and only after food during the day. Uncomfortable distension of abdomen, with a desire to belch up, not better by eructation. The periodicity of China still persists when the pain in the liver recurs periodically. The abdominal flatulence is present and feels better on bending double.

Hydrastis canadensis: there is gastro-duodenal catarrh, loud rumbling with dull aching, worse on moving. Sharp pain in the coecal area, and the spleen, and griping pain with the stool. There is jaundice torpor of the liver, with pale and scanty stools, pain in the liver extending to the back to the right scapula, while lying on the back. The liver is atrophied.

Phosphorus: it belongs to Tubercular constitution, nervous and weak person but intelligent. Burning is the character, craves icecream and cold things, chocolate, and salt. The liver is congested, jaundice with acute hepatitis. Has very foetid stools, with flatus, great weakness after the stool. Lot of belching, and throws up food by mouthful.

The treatment of cirrhosis is mainly palliative and the damage done to the liver cell is not reversible. But the progression may be halted by correcting the underlying cause.

Rest in bed is essential till the improvement continues.

Diet should be low in salt. Total intake should be about 2,000 cal, with protein intake of 120 gms. Fats and carbohydrate in normal quantity. Plenty of Vitamin B complex. Iron deficiency, anaemia should be treated through haematinics, B_{12} and folic acid. Milk should be restricted .Alcohol to be stopped.

Initially the treatment will be mostly symptomatic, depending on the case, and care should taken to avoid any complications.

25. ***Patient complains of pain in the gall bladder area, and the pain is paroxysmal, or dull or continuous and radiates to the right shoulder. There is tenderness in the gall bladder, vomiting and some fever. The disease is called*** *ACUTE CHOLECYSTITIS*.

The condition is very clear, one can feel the tender and enlarged gall bladder if the muscles are relaxed. The causes are stagnation of bile, calculi of solitary cholesterol type , foreign bodies like worms and ova, and the exciting cause can be any infection.

Cholesterinum: In such conditions where the diagnosis is in doubt, especially when the patient has been subjected to frequent biliary attacks, hepatic engorgement, and with or without jaundice. This remedy is almost specific. Burnett uses this in low potency of 3c.

Chionanthus virginica: acts powerfully on the liver, and gall bladder. This is a remedy for those living in malarial districts. Bilious colic, enormous liver, constipation and clay coloured stools, skin is yellow. Jaundice developing every summer. Abdominal pains are better by lying on abdomen. This remedy is useful in mother tincture and first potency.

Chelidonium maj: acts on the liver, portal system, right side of abdomen and right lower lung. Liver pains travel backwards and jaundice is developed due to hepatic and gall bladder obstruction. Prefers hot food and drink. Gastric pains are better after eating. There is decided aversion to cheese. Lower potencies are useful.

Berberis vulgaris: is useful in gall bladder colic as well as kidney colic. It promotes the flow of bile, the liver function is good but there is very little endurance. Sticking pain in the liver and gall bladder, shooting up the shoulder, worse by pressure. Jaundice follows the gall stone colic. Shooting pressure in the gall bladder area, worse from extending to stomach. Hard ball like stool, with constipation and yellow complexion.

26. ***An elderly female is suddenly seized with paroxysms of severe pain, in the hepatic region and in course of twelve to twenty-four hours, she becomes jaundiced, the stool becomes clay coloured. The attack is of BILIARY COLIC.***

Cholelithiasis is a condition when the gall stones are formed in the gall bladder. And the biliary colic is caused when the gall stones move along the ducts. When the stones are at rest there may not be any pain, but when they start moving there is agonizing pain — it starts in the epigastrium and shoots in the hypochondrium, towards the spine and up towards the right shoulder. These attacks are at times extremely severe. The symptoms arise of depending on position of the stone in the biliary tree.

Apart from the remedies which act on the pathology of gall bladder including the pain and colic, like Bell., Berberis vul., Carduus m., China, and cholesterinum, there are general colic drugs which have shown good results in gall stone colic.

Colocynthis: The characteristic griping pain in abdomen causes the patient to double up and this may accompany by colics in other parts of the body. Also, if stool occurs there is immediate relief. The pains come in waves and are better by doubling up and hard pressure. And is worse by eating or drinking.

Dioscorea : It is a remedy for many kinds of pains that dart about or radiate to distant parts. The pains and colic are unbearable, sharp, cutting, twisting, griping, and grinding. There are sharp pains in the liver shooting upwards to the nipple.

Morgan bacillus: Morgan bacillus is a bowel nosode. There are two sub-types — *Morgan Pure* and *Morgan Gaertner*. The key note of Morgan is congestion. There is epigastric pain or discomfort. There is pain in the liver and gall bladder, congestion of liver with bilious attacks. Severe headache, relieved with vomiting, there is recurrent bouts of indigestion.

4 FEMALE REPRODUCTIVE SYSTEM

- Primary and secondary amenorrhoea
- Dysmenorrhoea: Spasmodic, congestive, membranous
- Vaginitis
- Cervicitis
- Endometriosis
- Menorrhagia
- Metrorrhagia
- Uterine fibroids
- Pregnancy
- Morning sickness
- Menopause
- Abortion
- Cancer cervix
- Acute salpingitis

Gynaecology is the term used to describe the functions and diseases of the female reproductive organs. It is important to consider the whole individual as well as the organs from which the symptoms appear to originate.

Many women do not like to discuss their gynaecological problems and if they do, they do it with shyness and with frank embarrassment. History taking is, therefore, difficult. It is advisable to have a lady assistant present at that time of case taking.

Many women approach the physician with disorders of menstruation. The most common disorders are: Amenorrhoea, Oligomenorrhoea, Dysmenorrhoea, Menorrhagia and Metrorrhagia.

In general, the conditions which cause Primary Amenorrhoea are congenital, while those causing secondary amenorrhoea are acquired:

Primary	Secondary	
Delayed menarchy	*Hypothalamus*	*Emotional disturbance* *Endocrine disorders* *Oral Contraceptives* *Rare syndromes*
Craniopharyngioma	*Ant. Pit. Gland*	*Post Partum hypopituitarism* *Pituitary tumours*
Gonadal dysgenesis	*Ovaries*	*Polycystic ovarian syndrome* *Premature ovarian failure* *Functioning ovarian tumours*
Congenital absence *Testicular feminization*	*Uterus*	*Intra-uterine adhesions*
Imperforate Vagina	*Vagina*	*Acquired vaginal stenosis*

A correct history and physical examination is necessary if any medicinal treatment is to be started. Remember amenorrhoea is a symptom and not a disease. A proper assessment can be done by elaborating on the Causation, Sensation, Modalities and Concomitants.

1. ***A young unmarried girl of 18 years of age is brought in by her mother with a complaint that she has never menstruated till this time. This condition is PRIMARY AMENORRHOEA* OR *PUBERTY AMENORRHOEA.***

Full history and the examination of the patient is necessary. Blood examination to rule out anaemia. Biochemistry of the blood to determine the hormonal levels, sonography to determine the ovarian anatomy should be performed. Gynaecologist should be consulted to examine for imperforate hymen.

Rare condition of congenital absence of uterus, and non-canalization of vagina, infantile uterus or undeveloped ovaries. The patient should be subjected to a physical examination from an expert gynaecologist to determine the exact situation of congenital state. It may be noted here that with the congenital problems like absence of organs nothing can be done medicinally. However, infantile uterus or undeveloped ovaries can be treated with anti-miasmatic and constitutional homoeopathic remedies. Failure to develop an organ will fall into syphilitic miasm and failure to function will be under sycotic miasm. Success will depend upon the development of other secondary sex characters like development of breast, pubic and under-arm hair etc.

It may be necessary to study the constitution of the individual.

Ignatia: this is adapted to sensitive, excitable, nervous temperamental patient. Women of easily excitable nature. Romantic, idealistic, and over-worked, fatigued. Suitable to person who has been starving either from want or other causes. Women with ill-effects of disappointed love, grief, worry, jealousy, and some old spinal injuries. Constantly frustrated having internal conflicts with herself and worse from consolation. Amenorrhoea is usually due to grief.

Sepia: Sepia is of a delicate constitution, irritable and faint from least exertion. A very loving lady and a woman of career. She loves a person or any item as long as she can carry on her vocation without any obstacle but if she is obstructed in her work she is a worse person to deal with. The most common conditions are never well since puberty, ill-effects of anger and vexation, blows, injuries, over-lifting, jar, getting wet, laundry work, boiled milk, fat, pork, tobacco, and rape. Aversion to family to those loved best, to sympathy and to company, yet dread to be alone. Loves to dance and excited during thunderstorm.

Pulsatilla: it is remedy for females, mild, gentle, plethoric, yielding disposition, who cry readily, and weep when talking. Nervous debility or anaemia, Menses get suppressed by getting the feet wet, Menses are often delayed at the time of puberty. Pulsatilla ranges over the whole sexual period from puberty to menopause.

Aurum met: amenorrhoea with great sadness, menses are too late or scanty or absent. Swelling of axillary glands before menses appear. Usually all uterine complaints are associated with depression, and tendency to suicide.

Senecio aureus: amenorrhoea of young girls, with backache. Premature or too profuse menses. Menses are suppressed or retarded with concomitant symptoms. Dropsy cough and backache. Urinary disturbances.

High potency preparations of these remedies can often effectively change the mental states, bringing back the normal physiologic states.

Thyroidinum: there is infantile wasting, and arrested development of children.

Amenorrhoea in young girls, with gnawing in the uterus. Thyroidinum is suited to phosphoric type of patients, who on general are hyperthyroid as well as carbonic type.

Lycopodium: Grauvogol's carbonitrogenoid constitution. Keen intellectually but of feeble muscular development and undernourished. Menses get suppressed for months and breast develop nosodities with stitching and aching pains, rawness of nipples.

Kali carb: it is suited to persons of soft tissue, with tendency to be fat. Ill-effects of suppressions of eruptions in childhood, and never well after pneumonia. Amenorrhoea, difficult first menses with chest complaint and ascites.

2. ***A young woman between 18 and 22 who was menstruating earlier regularly reports —following a change in abode, or mode of life — anxiety, stress and mental shock. SECONDARY AMENORRHOEA.***

It is common in young girls who leave their homes say for studies or jobs. This anxiety and the fear of being alone, on one's own and that loss of protection for the first time outside the house can bring on changes in the hormonal balance that may cause the sudden cessation of the menses. There may not be any more symptoms except the absence of menses with slight heaviness in the head and congestive feeling. A timely administration of Aconite at times aided by Belladonna and Glonoinum will bring on the flow.

Aconite: Aconite has a nervous constitution, and have great fear and anxiety. Forebodings and fears are often present. Menses get suppressed because of fright.

Aconites are plethoric subjects and they may have very sudden menstrual bleeding and become frenzy, or there is sudden suppression of menses, which brings on fear and fright.

Glonoinum: It is suited to florid, plethoric, sensitive females, nervous, sanguine and readily affected persons. Complaints are brought on by ill-effects of sun, heat, bright snow, fire heat, fear or fright. Causes sudden cessation of menses with congestion to head. But in case this time is over more direct acting remedy may be required.

Pulsatilla: amenorrhoea from getting feet wet, nervous debility, anaemia. When prescribed between the intervals, 6th and 12th potency or five drops of mother tincture may bring on the flow. The alternate remedies may be Senecio and cyclamen if Pulsatilla fails.

Senecio aureus: it has some tonic effect on the general health. There is amenorrhoea in young girls with backache. Menses are retarded, suppressed with concomitant symptoms like dropsy, cough or backache. It is observed that there is nose-bleed or nasal catarrh, takes the place of menses when suppressed from any cause. .One more important use of this remedy is in condition where the condition is traceable to non-appearing menses.

Cyclamen: It is suited to blond leucophlegmatic subjects with chlorotic condition, disinclined for labour, and getting easily fatigued. Has changeable menses, suppression of menses after excessive dancing, or being overheated.

It will be necessary to restore the general health of the patient. Should this happen frequently due to derangement of health one will need to bring the necessary normalcy changes in health. Anemia is the most important cause.

Graphites: is indicated in defective menstruation with costiveness and tendency to skin eruption are a special indication, which forms the key-note. Very scanty menses — as good as nothing, when found with other complaints such as headaches, skin affection, moist itching excoriations and fissures.

Sepia: is most useful when there is leucorrhoea and portal and pelvic congestion with complains that she has never been well after puberty.

Sulphur: has scrofulous or unhealthy constitution with tendency to papular eruption or temporary congestions or flushes.

Natrum mur: has delayed first menstruation, constipation among its indication. Impaired nutrition and very dry skin. Headaches that are better after sleep.

Ignatia: very sensitive and excitable and nervous. Ill-effects of disappointed love, grief, worry and jealousy.

3. ***Patient is between 16 and 30 years of age and complains of severe pain at onset of the menstruation. This condition is probably SPASMODIC DYSMENORRHOEA.***

Many women experience this spasmodic pain or discomfort at the onset of menstruation, usually during the first few hours or the first day. The pain resembles colic. It accompanies vomiting, headache and malaise. This pain is usually at the sacrum or the left pelvic region and refers down into the legs. This often comes in patients with sedentary office-work or having no exercise. There is hardly any evidence of pelvic pathology. It is believed that the pain occurs because of the powerful uterine contractions which occur during the early days of the menstruation. Childbirth often cures this condition because the parous uterus is more vascular and more liable to become ischaemic.

Belladonna: suited to plethoric persons with red face and to conditions to where there is local plethora with pain, redness, throbbing, shining. The effects are very sudden. Violent burning heat, the pains are throbbing and cutting, neuralgic pains that come and go. Menses are bright red, too early and too profuse and are offensive, hot.

Mag phos: severe pains, neuralgic, they come and go along the course of the nerve, and these are better by hot application, pressure and bending double. Periodicity is another character.

Caulophyllum: is spasmodic and congestive for the first two days of the flow. Intermittent nature is characteristic. Menses are scanty preceded by severe pain in the small of the back. The pains fly in all directions. There is retroverted uterus, and irritable vagina. Rheumatism of small joints often is the concomitant symptom.

Cimicifuga: it causes depression of mind, with low spirits. The pains start in the ovarian region shoot upwards and down the anterior part of the thigh. Pain across the hip, hip to hip. These pains are just before the menses start flowing. Hysteric or epileptic spasms at the time of menses.Uterine atony. Leucorrhoea with sensation of weight in the uterus.

Gelsemium: the pains are with scanty flow, the pains extend to the back and hip; rigidity of the os with uterine inertia.

Sabina: suited to chronic ailments of women with arthritic pains, has a penetrating pain from the sacrum to pubes, Atony of the uterus with partly clotted haemorrhage. Worse from least motion. Dysmenorrhoea is better by lying flat on the bed with limbs extended. Shooting pains up the vagina.

Vibernum: is useful both in spasmodic and membranous dysmenorrhoea. Heavy aching feeling or excruciating cramps in the pelvis and this pain is better after menses appear. The pains then go around the waist. Sick feeling all over, in connection with the pelvic complaints and worse from movements, better by rest are key-notes of Vibernum.

Xanthoxyllum: is useful particularly in nervous person. The pains are almost agonizing along the course of the genito-crural nerve. Patient desires to take deep breath during the pains, with sensation of weakness in lower limbs. Menses are thick black. Ovarian neuralgia with pain in the loins and lower abdomen, worse on the left side, extending down the thigh, associated with neuralgic dysmenorrhoea, and neuralgic backache.

4. ***The patient is between 30 and 40 years of age and complains of pain several days before the menstruation . The condition may be CONGESTIVE DYSMENORRHOEA.***

The pains usually begin three or four days or up to a week before menstruation and it may be relieved or aggravated at its onset. The pain is felt in the pelvis or in the back. Exercise, movements aggravate it whereas the rest will ameliorate the pains.

Other conditions like menorrhagia, infertility or dysparunia are often associated with it. Chronic salpingitis and pelvic endometriosis are the main causes of this condition. Pelvic diathermy often relieves.

Sabina: has a very characteristic pain, sacrum to pubis, pain before the flow starts. Dysmenorrhoea, better lying flat on the back with limbs extended. Menses are too profuse and too early, gushing of hot water. Bright blood mixed with dark clots, pains from sacrum to pubis and from below upwards. Belladonna has hot haemorrhage, breast pains are worse lying down, throbbing pains, bright red, too early and too profuse.

Viburnum op.: has great sickly feeling with pain in the back going around the loin and to pubic bones: with bearing down sensation, relieved from lying down and aggravated by movements. Mother tincture in drop doses seem to act better.

Secale cor: menses are irregular, copious, dark fluid, accompanied by labour-like pains in abdomen, and continuous watery discharge of blood, during the whole time between the periods. In potencies seem to be effective and is beneficial when prescribed in between the periods.

5. ***A woman between the age of 15 and 45 complains of very severe pain at the onset of menstruation which is relieved by the passage of casts (clots). The condition is MEMBRANOUS DYSMENORRHOEA.***

This condition can occur at every cycle or at occasional cycles. A portion or the complete cast of the endometrium can pass with pain. The pain is due to contraction of the uterus. Initially the bleeding may be scanty, may increase with the passage of cast.

Belladonna: has throbbing pains and accompanied by red bright blood with severe pains from hip to hip. The pains come suddenly and go suddenly.

Hamamelis: is useful for vicarious menstruation. Menses are dark profuse, with soreness in abdomen. Bleeding at times is between periods. Ovarian congestion and neuralgia.

Chamomilla: with the uterine pain if there is increased tension and irritability of mind with very uncivil attitude, more so at puberty. Profuse oozing of dark foul blood, with black clots with coldness of limbs and much thirst.

Coffea: has neuralgia and sensitivity of every part with great excitability and intolerance of pain driving to despair, toothache during menses. Voluptuous itching in the vulva, very sensitive and therefore aversion to sex.

6. ***There is a thin non-purulent discharge from vulval orifice, the condition is LEUCORRHOEA.***

A small amount of secretion is healthy. This secretion tends to increase before ovulation and menstruation in normal women. It is a non-infective type of discharge and is an increase in the normal secretion of the genital tract.

It is common at puberty, ovulation and before the onset of menstruation, increases with sexual excitement, during pregnancy. May accompany local congestion due to overexertion, constipation or gastroenteritis and other causes of pelvic congestion. Debility, anaemia and malnutrition. Cervical erosion is most common cause of this discharge — mostly in young.

It is necessary to remove any local cause : Pay attention to the health. Advise fresh air and exercise and general tonic treatment.

Since the discharge is different in terms of consistency, colour, odour, time of flow, concomitant symptoms, the remedies also differ. Nevertheless, in our day-to-day practice we use some remedies which are indicated again and again.

One must understand that leucorrhoea is not a disease by itself but a symptom and may be associated with other uterine maladies. Leucorrhoea occurrs with general debility which we find mostly in the tropical countries like ours, over lactation. Here, apart from improving the general state of patient can consider **Helonias diosca:** which has strong action on the uterus. It is a great uterine tonic. Its characteristic symptom is "consciousness of the womb". There is uterine displacement because of the generalized weakness. There is intense pruritus of the vulva and pudenda and there is thin discharge. The patient is lethargic and slow in its work.

Pulsatilla: is another very important remedy when Helonias seem not to work. The remedy is sort of specific. Leucorrhoea following abortions, or after bearing children too often, with the congestion of the womb.

Sabina and **Sepia:** are chief remedies for leucorrhoea following abortions or after bearing children with the congestion of the womb. The leucorrhoea is profuse, milky, starchy, ropy, with drawing pains in the broad of the back in Sabina.

Sepia: is never well since puberty, childbirth, after weaning or after getting off the hormone pills. Leucorrhoea is yellow, greenish, milky, in large lumps in little girls in place of menses; there is constant bearing down sensation as if the entire contents of the pelvis will come out. When the discharge degenerates into an acrid and offensive fluid low potency works better.

Kreosote: will be the remedy of choice when the discharge degenerates to an acrid offensive fluid, there is erosion of cervix, stitches in vagina, menses are too early and prolonged. Haemorrhage or violent pains, during and after sex, burning in parts after sex, followed by discharge of dark blood the next day. Often there is some malignancy in the uterus.

7. ***Patient complains of a purulent discharge coming from the vagina, the condition is VAGINITIS.***

This condition can be acute or chronic. In acute condition the discharge is profuse, yellow or greenish, sometimes it is blood-stained, attended by dysuria, and local signs of inflammation.

The main causes are trauma, foreign bodies, and worms in children, in adult can be irritant pessary, tampoon and or excessive coitus, specific or non-specific infection, extension of infection from adjacent organs, urethra or bartholin gland.

Prior to the medicinal treatment cleaning of vagina with speculum and Calendula 1 : 10 aqueous solution is a good practice. In children, this cleansing is necessary under general anaesthesia.

Belladonna is suited to plethoric patients, red face and to conditions where there is local plethora, an inflammatory state with pain throbbing and shiny redness. Dryness and heat in the vagina, the discharges are badly smelling.

Hydrastis is useful in older and easily tired people, cachectic individuals with great debility and emaciation. Erosion and excoriation of cervix, thick yellow ropy leucorrhoea, pruritus vulvae with profuse leucorrhoea, discharge after menses which is acrid and corroding, shreddy, tenacious, with sexual excitement.

Caladium: has a marked action on the genital organs. And itching in this region. Itching of vulva and vagina, voluptuous and itching leads to masturbation. There is burning and cramp-like pains in the uterus at night.

Cannabis sativa: it affects specially the urinary and sexual organs. Acute and chronic gonorrhoea. There is inflammatory state making the patient walk with legs apart. Threatened abortion with too frequent intercourse. Conditions following acute gonorrhoea, miscarriage. Great sexual excitement with infertility.

Cantharis : there is constant discharge from the vagina aggravated by false step, associated with cystitis, black swelling of the vulva, and burning pain in the ovaries. There is dragging pain in the sacrum usually after a miscarriage, with too frequent and profuse menses, leucorrhoea, swollen and tender breast.

Helonias : menses are suppressed, parts are hot red swollen with loss of sexual desire. They burn and itch terribly.

Kreosote: there is yellow acrid discharge having an odour of green corn that is worse between the periods.

Medorrhinum: there is intense itching in the vagina better by rubbing, and by bathing in tepid water. Sycotic warts on genitals, ovarian pain on the left side, or from ovary to ovary. The menses are profuse and dark, offensive stains are difficult to wash. Medorrhinum is usually given in single dose in the acute stages of the disease.

Thuja: menses are too early and short, scanty and retarded. Lot of itching in the vagina, profuse leucorrhoea, thick, greenish with cauliflower-like excrescences. Vagina is very sensitive that prevents sex. Polyps and fleshy excrescences.

Staphysagria: painful and sensitive genitals, worse sitting down, First sex is very painful, causing acute bodily and mental agony, granular growth of vagina. History of rape, sexual-abuse victim.

Platina: patient has painful sensitive genitals, with itching, tickling and crawling sensation. Excessive sexual desire. Dark clotted too early menses.The organs are very sensitive inducing the masturbation. But sex is impossible.

8. ***Middle-aged married lady complains of constant vaginal discharge — glary material like white of an egg, at times it is muco-purulent. In addition to this discharge there is backache, pelvic or lower abdominal pain, The condition is CERVICITIS.***

Nitric Acid: there are stitches through the vagina. Voluptuous itching in the vagina after sex. Leucorrhoea is brown, flesh coloured, watery or stringy, stains yellow or leaves spots, with black border. Bloody water from vagina, or haemorrhage from over-exertion. Uterine haemorrhage after child-birth or curetting.

Alumen: induration of cervix. Menses are scanty, watery. Left ovary is affected. Chronic gonorrhoeal discharge, with little lumps along the urethra. Vagina is very sensitive, and narrowed by swellings. Itching with aphthous patch in the vagina.

Kali Bichrom: adapted to fat, fair, flabby, fleshy, person, subject to catarrhs with syphilitic or scrofulous history. Mostly overweight person. Menses are suppressed or red urine. Leucorrhoea is yellow acrid, ropy with pain across sacrum,and heaviness in the hypogastrium. Prolapse uterus in hot weather. Itching and burning of the vulva with sexual excitement. Pruritus vulvae with great burning and excitement. The ulcers are characteristic with punched out margins but regular, with stringy mucous discharge.

Ustilago maydis: adapted to tall and thin women usually at menopause. Uterine fibroids, bleeding with hypertrophy of the uterus. Cervix is spongy and bleeds easily. Menses are half liquid and half clotted, bright red and worse on slightest provocation. Foul yellow or brown leucorrhoea. Uterus feels as if drawn into knots. Low potency repeated is more useful.

9. ***Elderly lady between 30 and 40 years of age with sterility and dysparunia, complains of pain before the onset of menstrual flow and may cause congestive dysmenorrhoea, the flow relieves the pain. The condition may be ENDOMETRIOSIS.***

Endometriosis is considered today as a very common disease of the pelvic organs in the females.

On examination and study of the case of endometriosis one will find that the lady occasionally complains of haematuria, depending on the situation of the growth. Fibroids are frequently detected, associated menorrhagia.

Treatment that is suggested in older women is usually surgical but in younger women conservative treatment at times suggested.

For homoeopathic treatment it is necessary to get the constitution of the patient.

Iodium: its action is mostly on the glands, thyroid, testes, mesentric and mammary.New growths and hyperplasia, and having fast growths. They have great weakness during menses, but it is irregular,brown in colour, renewed after every stool, wedge-like pain from ovary to uterus, in the right ovarian area. Ovaritis, Leucorrhoea is acrid, eroding thighs, and linen. Sterility from atrophy of ovaries.

Palladium: it affects the right ovaries, uterus and mind. Being an ovarian remedy it causes symptom complex of Oophoritis. Pains are fleeting and transient. Pains in the right ovary are better by pressure. Subacute pelvic peritonitis, with menorrhagia. Uterine prolapse with retro-version, cutting pains in the uterus, relieved after stool. Shooting and burning pain in the pelvis, bearing down pains better by rubbing. Soreness and shooting pains from navel to breast. Glarey yellow leucorrhoea, before and after menses.

Sabina: it is a remedy for the chronic ailments of women, arthritic pains, tendency to miscarriage, and gouty diathesis. Women particularly with haemorrhagic tendency and nose-bleeds. Tendency to miscarriage, especially at the third month. Dysmenorrhoea better lying down flat on the bed, with limbs extended. Dark blood clots with bright bleeding. Uterine pains extend into the thighs. Increased desire for sex. Shooting pains in the vagina. Discharge of blood in between the periods.

Secale cor: the constitution is that of haemorrhagic diathesis. Weak uterus or bearing down pains with coldness. Passive haemorrhage with hour-glass contraction.

Brownish offensive leucorrhoea. Threatened abortion by about the third month. Although cold, aggravated by external heat.

Pulsatilla: it is a remedy for mild, gentle, plethoric, yeilding, dispositioned female who would cry easily while talking. Three characteristics: chilly, worst by warmth and thirstless — must be present for this remedy. In the female, pulsatilla ranges over the whole sexual period — from puberty to the menopause. Including menstruation, pegnancy, and breast-feeding.

10. ***A middle-aged woman complains of excessive bleeding during the menstrual flow. The condition is MENORRHAGIA.***

After taking the history proceed to examine the various causes of bleeding in the individual. There may be local causes or constitutional causes.

Normal menstruation varies from one woman to other. Some women have profuse bleeding at every menstrual cycle all their life. They are plethoric and have florid countenances. Excessive menstruation may be due to hypertension, too many and too frequent pregnancies and prolonged lactation, acute specific fevers, sepsis or purpura, endocrine imbalance, as at puberty.

Belladonna: suited to plethoric persons, with red face and local plethora. Ill-effects of hair getting wet, sunstroke, walking in the wind or draft. Fullness and congestion especially to head, throbbing and are other characters of the drug. Basically a chilly person and expresses violence in every symptom. Menses are bright red sand, excessive, offensive and hot. Worse from heat of the sun, and after heated with the drafts of wind. Worse at night.

Phosphorus: Phosphorus stands at the head of the haemorrhagic remedies. The blood loses its coagubility, and even the slightest wound bleeds. The menses are too profuse, longer lasting than usual. There can be vicarious menstruation in the form of haemoptysis, nose bleed or haematuria. Sometimes there is no profuse bleeding but they last long. There is a possibility of infertility with this profuse bleeding.

Ipecacuanha: it is particularly suited to women of emphysematous state with frequent nose bleed.The uterine haemorrhage is bright red, steady flow, or gushing with nausea, gasping with each gush of blood. At times there may be prolapse of the uterus with profuse bleeding.

Sabina: suited to plethoric women who suffer from rheumatic inflammation. Suited to hot-blooded women with gouty and rheumatic diathesis. Haemorrhagic tendency, Haematuria Menses are too profuse and early gushing hot, mixed with clots, uterine pain extends into thighs, pains from sacrum to pubis, shooting pain in the vagina.

11. ***An elderly lady gives history of irregular haemorrhage from the uterus irrespective of the menstrual period. The condition is METRORRHAGIA.***

Uterine bleeding is covered by many drugs. Most important are the constitutional remedies having marked action on the physiology of the uterus.

Calcarea carb: deep antipsoric constitutional remedy, Scrofulous type taking cold easily. Leuco-phlegmatic temperament and the disorders are caused by working for long hours in water. The menses are too early, too profuse and too long. Mental excitement causes the menses to return, at times with dysmenorrhoea.

Belladonna: is acute of Calcarea and often has the violent bleeding with throbbing. Bright red blood; too early and too profuse.

China officinalis: China is suited to persons of thin, dry, bilious constitution. Leucophlegmatic person. Menses are too early, dark, profuse, clotted, with abdominal distension. Bloody leucorrhoea seems to take place of menses of the usual menstrual discharge.

Crocus sativa: suited to women with hysterical tendencies. Crocus has three characteristics: Haemorrhage from any outlet, where the blood is black and stringy, clotting and forming into long string hanging from the bleeding orifice. Worse from the least movement.

Hamamelis: person with venous constitution. Menses are dark, profuse, with soreness in the abdomen. Jolting brings on menstrual bleeding. Bleeding midway between the menstrual periods only in the daytime, intermenstrual pains, ovarian congestions and neuralgia, feels very sore.

Lachesis: women nearing menopause. Symptoms like palpitation, hot flushes, haemorrhage vertex and headaches. Menses are too short and too feeble with uterine and ovarian pains relieved by the flow. They are black, scanty, lumpy, more of pain and less of flow.

Millefolium: is suited to aged, atonic, anaemic women. Useful in prolonged bleeding, of a hard labour. Menses are early, profusely protracted. Heamorrhages are bright red fluid. Suppressed menstruation with epileptic attacks.

This is not the complete list, many other remedies can be considered. Here the constitution of the patient is more important.

In both the above cases it will be necessary to keep watch on the anaemia of the patient. And replenish the same by giving iron and calcium and multivitamins.

12. ***An elderly patient gives history of excessive bleeding, heaviness of abdomen at the time of menstruation and at times otherwise also. Sometimes this bleeding is associated with severe pain. The case is of a** UTERINE FIBROID.*

The uterine fibroids may be submucous, interstitial or subserous. When the fibroid is submucous or interstitial, the symptoms are menorrhagia or metrorrhagia, and at times there is dysmenorrhoea. Examination will show that there is enlarged uterine cavity and bimanual examination may reveal bossed and hard mass of fibroids. The subserous fibroids may present no symptoms for many years and may be detected by accident. Some pressure symptoms may be present. Large fibroids will undergo degeneration and will give rise to pain and symptoms of toxaemia.

At present the newer techniques of imaging and that of sonography can show the presence of fibroids in a early stage. The medical treatment is possible if detected at the beginning of the process. But later, only solution is surgical removal of these fibroids.

In homoeopathy we depend on our constitutional remedies and on the acute remedies depending on the presentation of signs and symptoms.

The submucous variety tends to become polypoid, remaining attached to the uterine wall by a pedicle. The subserous presents no symptoms for many years, and is discovered by accident. Pressure symptoms are its earliest symptoms. In these uterine fibroids the growth rate is most individual.

Fraxinus americana: it is an uterine tonic for nervous females. Especially with fibroids, with bearing-down sensation, cramping in feet. Uterus is enlarged, heavy and prolapsed. Watery non-irritating leucorrhoea. There is profuse menstrual bleeding with sensitive left ovary.

Lilium tigrinum: there is prolapse or anteverted uterus. Menses are early, scanty and dark. Clotted offensive. Flow only when moving about. There is constant desire to support the parts externally. Cannot bear the pressure of clothes.

Ustilago: its use at menopause more in tall, thin, women. Uterine fibroids bleeding, hypertrophy of the uterus, sub-involution. Cervix is spongy and bleeds easily, half clotted and half liquid, bright red, worse on slightest provocation.

Thlaspi bursa pastoris: it is remedy of haemorrhages and uric acid diathesis. Uterine haemorrhages are with cramps and expulsion of clots. Metrorrhagia too frequent and copious menses. Every alternate period is very profuse. Leucorrhoea before and after menses. Stains are indelible, sore pain in the womb on rising. Scarsely recover from one period before another begins.

Trillium pendulum: suited to women who bleed after labour pain. Menses every two weeks. Uterine haemorrhage with sensation as though hips and back were falling apart to pieces, better on tight bandaging. Least movement renews the bleeding. Haemorrhages from the fibroids.

Aurum muriaticum natronatum : this double salt of Natrum and chloride of Gold shows more of presence of syphilitic miasm. Burnett states that there is no other powerful remedy over uterine tumours than this. It has induration of one part and softening of the other. Its action is primarily on the uterus and the ovaries and the breast. There is chronic metritis and prolapsed uterus.

Calcarea flouricum: is a very powerful tissue remedy for hard stony glands, varicose veins and malnutrition of bones. In females, there is excessive bleeding, with prolapsed uterus, dragging down sensation in uterus and thighs.

13. ***A recently married woman staying with her husband complains of severe nausea and vomiting on waking up and that she had not had her periods since last two months. The condition is probably PREGNANCY VOMITING or MORNING SICKNESS.***

Pregnancy is normal physiological phenomenon and amenorrhoea following that pregnancy is the earliest sign of pregnancy. In some women they show signs of early morning vomiting.

Nux vom: this is the first of the remedies to be thought of. There is irritability, hiccough from over-eating, morning sickness, varicose veins, and haemorrhoids. False labour pains. Sensation of indigestion. Flatulence and heart-burn, sour bitter belching.

Ipecac: constant nausea and vomiting, not better by vomiting, nausea with copious salivation. Retching, especially after drinking anything cold or after smoking.

Symphoricarpus racemosa: it is highly recommended for persistent nausea and vomiting of pregnancy. Worse from any motion. Averse to all type of food, better when lying on the back. Smell and thought of food repugnant.

Lactic acid: a very valuable remedy in morning sickness in anaemic pale women. Water brash is better after breakfast.

Sepia: bloating of abdomen with acid dyspepsia and sour belching. Boiled milk disagrees. Faint sinking feeling in the epigastrium not better by eating. Belching of milk, sour bitter, rancid of tough, foamy mucus. Nausea at the sight or thought of food in the morning.

In fact, no treatment is necessary for this condition unless the whole nausea and vomiting episodes cause constitutional symptoms endangering the pregnancy. Management of these morning sickness patient is important.

Patient should be advised complete rest in bed, on waking up and without getting up she should rinse the mouth at the bedside, and should eat dry crackers or salted biscuits or some sweet like bread and jam, or any home-made sweet preparation and no water or tea should be taken for at least half hour. This normally settles down that nauseating feeling. Small helpings of food should be suggested at frequent intervals, lots of fruits and fruit juices should be encouraged. Bed rest initially in the morning and normal activity in the house can be advised.

14. ***An elderly female of 50 years age complains of hot flushes, sometimes accompanied by sweating, insomnia, irritability, depression and restlessness, and that she has been experiencing delayed and irregular menstruation over the last one year or so most probably she is attaining MENOPAUSE.***

Menopause is the epoch in a woman at which the reproductive activity of the female undergoes involution and the menses which are the sign of that activity cease. The signs and symptoms are the one mentioned by the patient, along with that the atrophic changes occur through out the genital organs, including the uterus which shrinks. There are various patterns of ceasation of this menstrual flow. It may disappear suddenly after the last period or it might linger every month for a longer time or have an excessive bleeding for a while and cease totally. This is the time when the patient experiences emotional disturbances, flushing of face, palpitation and as if ants are crawling under the skin. These episodes last for few minutes. Normally, between the age of 15 to 35 even though the vaginal opening, urethral opening and the rectum are very close to each other, incidence of urinary infection is very less because of healthy endothelial lining and natural immunity. But after menopause there is atrophy of endothelial lining and urinary infection, vaginal infection , fungal infection become very common. So these conditions need attention.

Graphites: menses are late, scanty, pale, irregular and painful. Swelling and hardness of the left ovary, worse after menses. There is induration of ovaries, uterus and breast. Vagina is dry hot and, at times, cold. There is aversion to sex.

Lachesis: menopausal complaints like palpitation, hot flushes, vertex headache, fainting spells, worse by pressure of clothes. Uterine and ovarian pains all are relieved after the flow sets in.

Manganum: the flushes of heat at menopause and discharge of blood in-between the periods. Their first menses are delayed, and scanty in anaemic patients.

Sepia : hot flushes with perspiration, bearing down sensation from vagina as if everything will fall down.

15. ***A married woman with about 22 weeks' pregnancy reports with slight bleeding per vagina but complains having no pains, it is probably a case of THREATENED ABORTION.***

Here the cervix is closed and the size if the uterus corresponds with the period of amenorrhoea, preceding the bleeding.

Viburnum opulus: suited to tall slender and fair-haired hysterical subject. It is remedy for general cramps, and colicky pains in the pelvic organs. It is claimed that it prevents miscarriages. Violent spasmodic nervous effects depending on the uterine or ovarian origin. Pains make her very nervous, and cannot keep still. She has spasmodic and membranous dysmenorrhoea. Uterine pains extend around the pelvis, often extending down the thighs. Pelvic organs feel as if turning upside down.

Sabina: it is suited to chronic ailments of women. Tendency to miscarriage. Plethoric women. Atony of the uterus, and uterine haemorrhage, partly clotted, worse from least motion. Tendency to miscarriage in the third month and menorrhagia in women who aborted readily. Pain in the sacrum to pubis and shooting pain up the vagina. Bleeding between the period with sexual excitement. Violent pulsation, wants windows open. There is sudden increase in the pains but they subside slowly.

Trillium pendulum: is suited to women who are flabby and bleed after every labour pain. It is a great haemorrhagic remedy, particularly uterine haemmorhage, often in threatened abortion, with cramp-like pains. There is a sensation as though hip and back falling to pieces, better tight bandages. Slightest movement induces gushing of blood. And there is flooding with fainting. It has been found useful and often curative in ante-partum, menopausal, in fibroid tumours and in haemorrhages of all kinds.

Secale cor: threatened miscarriage takes place about the third month. There are severe after-pains. The uterus is weak, or having bearing down pain. Contracted uterus, or hour-glass contraction. Haemorrhage is passive with burning pain in the uterus. Though the patient is cold to touch does not bear to be covered. And in spite of this coldness, Secale has burning among the characteristic sensations. Worse by external heat.

Sepia: has tendency to miscarriage from fifth to seventh month. There is severe itching in the vulva causing abortion. Sepia is one who is never well after puberty, or a child-birth, or after weaning, or stopping the hormone pills. Uterus is weak and constant dragging down sensation. There is griping sticking or burning in uterus. After abortion there is, at times, retained placenta.

Erigeron: Erigeron has been an haemorrhagic remedy with profuse, bright red, gushing and persistent haemorrhage even from the bladder. Exertion causes miscarriage. Pregnant women with weak uterus, and a bloody discharge on slight exertion.

Croccus sativa: three important characteristics are when haemorrhage is black, dark, stringy, clotting, forming into long black strings hanging from the bleeding orifice. Peculiar sensations as if something alive was moving in the abdomen. Rapid changes of sides of the symptoms, or alternate with mental and physical symptoms.

Caulophyllum: Acts most markedly on the female degenerative organs and the rheumatic state. It is a woman's remedy and there is lack of tone of the uterus, left ovarian and infra breast pains. There is habitual miscarriage due to uterine debility. The labour pains are weak or irregular, and there are false labour pains. Extraordinary rigidity of the os .Lochia is profuse and prolonged. The labour pains and small joint pains alternate.

16. ***A middle-aged multiparus woman complains of excessive bleeding during the menstrual period and also in-between the period, and intervening period there is pinkish brown discharge with offensive odour and also complains of slight bleeding on exertion and coitus.***

It is a case of CANCER OF CERVIX

Carcinoma cervix runs a variable course but its progress is more rapid in younger women. When the patient comes with above complaints, in the early stages the os feels hard, friable, and granular and the examining fingers will be blood-stained and at the later stages will reveal mushroom-like growth, rapidly breaking-down and bleeding. But the local pains are usually late. Early diagnosis helps the patient to survive.

Conium mac: Corresponds to old feeble patients, patients with strong sedentary habits, those easily getting intoxicated with stimulants, cancerous diathesis with glandular enlargements. They are of scrofulous constitution. Menses are too late and scanty. Itching around pudenda or deep in the vagina. Has signs of cervicitis, induration of os and cervix. It has unsatisfactory and ill-effects of repressed sexual desires, or suppressed menses due to excessive indulgence.

Aurum met: Menses are too late and scanty or absent. Uterus gets enlarged and there is prolapse. There is mental depression because of frequent miscarriages and barrenness that follows; has a tendency to suicide. The leucorrhoea is profuse and corroding, yellow thick white.

Carbo animalis: It is suited to greatly debilitated and of feeble constitution. Menses are too early, frequent and long-lasting, dark clotted putrid flow. With the cancer of the uterus, burning pain down the thighs, pelvic bones, pain on sitting. Indurated os with burning. Even the breast gets affected darting painful indurations.

Kreosotum: Menses are profuse, lumpy, corrosive itching within vulva, the menses flow intermittently, cease on sitting or walking. Burning soreness in external or internal parts. Cancer of the uterus or with erosion of cervix. Haemorrhage after sex, violent pain during sex, followed by discharge of dark blood next day.

Hydrastis canadensis: There is thick yellow ropy, profuse leucorrhoea, with pruritus vulvae. There is erosion and excoriation of cervix, vagina sore during coitus; bleeding afterwards, hot watery discharge from the uterus. Indicated also in fibroid tumours at menopause. Menorrhagia and metrorrhagia with fibroids.

Ustilago maydis: There is uterine bleeding due to fibroids, and hypertrophy of the uterus. Cervix is spongy which easily bleed. Half clotted, half bright red, worse on slightest provocation. Uterus feels as if drawn into knots.

17. ***A female patient complains of severe pain across the lower abdomen, with distension, tenderness and rigidity. There is temperature with quick pulse. The condition may be ACUTE SALPINGITIS.***

The commonest result of acute pelvic inflammation is acute salpingitis. Apart from the symptoms the patient describes, there is great tenderness and pain on moving the cervix during bimanual examination. There is often bleeding or muco-purulent discharge from the cervix.

Arsenic alb: There is burning in the ovarian region: pressive, stretching pains in ovary into the thigh, which feels numb and lame, worse on motion or bending. The pains are often better by warm application.

Apis : There is soreness and stinging pains — mostly in the right ovary. Ovaries are numb and congested with suppressed menses. The pains in the ovaries are worse on sex. There is great tenderness over the abdomen and uterine region. Amenorrhoea at puberty.

Colocynthis: Dysmenorrhoea, worse eating and drinking. Boring pains in ovary and must bend over double with great restlessness. Clutching pains in the ovarian region. Ovarian tumours or cysts in ovaries and broad ligament. Pain better by flexing the legs.

Medorrhinum: it is a great ant-sycotic remedy. Ovarian pains are worse in the left side and from ovary to ovary. There is intense menstrual colic. Metrorrhagia, menses are offensive, profuse, dark, clotted stains are difficult to wash out. There is sensitive spot near the os uterus.

Sepia : it causes engorgement of the uterus which turns into induration. Offensive yellowish green leucorrhoea, with either prolapse or retroversion. There is constant sense of pressing in the vagina. With this symptom of pelvic bearing down, and connected with these uterine symptoms are hysteria, palpitation, orgasm of the blood and faintness.

18. ***Females, usually after 30, complains of profound depression, irritability, emotional outbursts, sometimes insomnia during 7 to 10 days before menstruation. There may also be weight gain, bloated feeling and pain in breasts. The condition is PREMENSTRUAL SYNDROME or PREMENSTRUAL TENSION.***

A proper case history taking is essential. Leading symptoms, nature of menstruation, character of earlier pregnancies, miscarriages, micturation, and, if married, dysparunia and any contraception being used should be inquired into.The treatment will depend on the acute symptoms presented by the patient. This is mostly sycopsoric state with superimposed tubercular state.

Calcarea carb: This an antipsoric constitutional remedy. Severe headache, colics, chilliness and leucorrhoea before menses. Mental excitement brings on dysmenorrhoea or causes menses to return. Breast swollen and tender menses. Hot swelling of the breast.

Calcarea Phos: The sexual organs are the center of many complaints. Nymphomania, with irresistible desire before menses. Voluptuous feeling, as all the parts were filled with blood. Pulses in all the parts with increased desire for urination.

Bovista: Has diarrhoea before and after menses. Menses are worse at night. There is acrid corrosive leucorrhoea.

Kali carb: Water retention, swollen breasts. Violent colicky pains before menses. Moods keep on changing, irritable and weeps, full of fear and imagination.

Lachesis: There are many complaints those start prior to menstrual flow, and get better after the flow sets in. All the uterine pains are better after the onset of menses. Breasts are affected. There are some obstinate eruption on the breast around the areola. This is useful, therefore, at the time of menopause.

Lac caninum: The breasts are swollen and painful before menses — relieved after the flow sets in. The flow is in gushes. There is symptom alternation from right to left.

Pulsatilla: Manic state before the menses. There is nose-bleed before and after suppressed menses.

5 KIDNEYS AND URINARY TRACT

- Acute Nephritis
- Urinary tract Infection
- Rena colic
- Retention of urine
- Nephrotic Syndrome
- Pyelonephritis
- Cystitis
- Urethritis
- Suppression of Urine

Throughout the urinary tract we find the latent symptoms of all miasms but psora and sycosis take active part in the production of disease in these organs. Not that the tubercular miasm is absent, we see its presence associated with sycotic elements in the production of malignancies and severe disease of this system. The tubercular and sycotic expressions are present in majority of inflammatory process like Acute nephritis.

1. ***The patient presents with illness of recent origin, with large quantity of albumen and tube casts passing in the urine, it is smoky to look at because of presence of blood, the condition is ACUTE NEPHRITIS.***

The main cause of this condition is streptococcus haemolyticus commonly found in tonsils. These can follow after an attack of influenza, typhoid, malaria, cerebrospinal fever, staphylococcus infection and trench fever. Sudden chilling can predispose. This usually terminates in recovery.

Apis Mellifica: the characteristic pathological state corresponds to Apis — Inflammation of the kidney, constricted sensation. Swelling or puffiness of various parts, oedema, red rosy.

Increased flow of urine shows a favourable effect. Dropsies of Apis are characterized by waxy hue of skin, whitish or transparent swelling of eyelids, bag-like swelling under the eyes.

Copaiva: there is burning pressure and painful urination by drops. Retention of urine with pain in the bladder, anus and rectum. Constant desire to urinate. Urine is acrid, scanty, bloody, odour of violet, greenish turbid colour, and peculiar pungent odour.

Terebinthina: it is for both acute and chronic nephritis. Main remedy where there is protein and blood in urine. Often the damage to the kidney is due to inhalation of chemicals. Burning is the main symptom. Often found useful when nephritis has developed after scarlatina and consequent dropsy in cases of albuminuria, and haematuria. The urine is smoky and turbid, and urine depositing sediment like grounded coffee.

Ocimum canum: pain in the kidney with violent vomiting.Right-sided kidney colic. Red urine with brick dust sediment after the attack. The urine may be saffron-coloured and thick, purulent with intolerable smell like musk. The patient has a uric acid diathesis. And red sand in urine is characteristic. Right-sided kidney colic. There is proteinuria, and thick urine.

Berberis vulgaris: the pains travel from kidney to the bladder. Bubbling sensation in the kidney. Frequent urination, dysuria, urethra burns when not urinating, urine is thick with red sand, turbid, yellow sandy and slimy urine. The pains radiate.

Cantharis: constant desire to urinate, cutting pains before and during urination. Sensitive kidney with dropsy. Urine is burning and scalding, with cutting pain and intolerable itching. Urine passes drop by drop, sometimes dribbling.

During the acute phase it will be necessary to reduce the load of work on the kidney by giving the maximum of fluids. Intake and output chart should be maintained. Blood pressure should be regularly monitored. The diet should be salt-free and low in proteins. Gradually carbohydrates might be added with increase in fluid content.

2. ***Patient is usually a female or a child complaining of frequency of micturition day and night with painful voiding, smelly urine, haematuria, and suprapubic pain and tenderness. It is a URINARY TRACT INFECTION.***

These symptoms relate to bladder and urethral inflammation commonly called cystitis, and suggest lower urinary tract infection.

Loin pain, tenderness, fever, and systemic upset suggest extension of the infection to the pelvis and kidney — known as pyelitis or pyelonephritis. Urinary tract infection can exist without any associated symptoms.

In children who cannot complain accurately their symptoms, their possibility of UTI is to be considered on the basis of their fretful febrile sickness, and who fail to thrive.

Cantharis: constant desire to urinate, intolerable tenesmus, cutting before, during, and after urination. Urine is burning, scalding with cutting pains, and intolerable urging. Urine is passed drop by drop, and atony of the bladder due to long retention of urine.

Apis: burning and soreness when urinating. Dysuria with stinging pain, last drops scald. The urine is loaded with casts and is albuminous. Stinging pain and strangury. Difficult and slow urine, and needs to press due to prostate affections.

Cannabis sativa: inflammed sensation with soreness to touch. Urethra is sensitive and walks with his legs apart. Must strain to urinate, and has to wait for some time before the urine starts flowing and dribbles after the flow ceases. Burning in the urethra extends to the bladder. There is zigzag pain in the urethra. Urine is turbid white, or reddish. Typically a sycotic remedy with gonorrhoeal infection.

Staphysagria: very important remedy for cystitis in young married women, often called honeymoon cystitis. There is pressure in the bladder, feels that it did not empty. Urinates into a thin stream or drop by drop. There is feeling of constant rolling of drop along urethra followed by burning in urethra. Burning in urethra when not urinating.

Ferrum picricum: pain along entire urethra, frequent urination, at night, with full feeling. Retention of urine. Smarting at the neck of the bladder and penis. Concomitant pressure in the rectum with constipation.

Sycotic bacillus: irritation of the mucus membrane from kidney to urethra. Frequency and urgency. Urine is corrosive. Urinary tantrums with pain in the kidney. This is a nosode (Bowel Nosode) prepared from the non-lactose fermenting cocci of the intestinal tract and, therefore, useful as inter-current remedy in Albuminuria, Nephritis, Nephrosis, Pyelitis, and Cystitis.

The pre-and post-treatment cultures are mandatory. In relapse a search should be made to find the cause. Reinfection implies that the patient has a poor defence system and prophylactic measures should be taken.

Fluid intake must increase to at least two liters. Instruction to void the urine every 2-3 hours should be given. Voiding of urine before bedtime and after intercourse. Patient be instructed to avoid bubble baths and chemical baths. And to avoid constipation.

3. ***Patient gives the history of severe paroxysms of lancinating pain, starting in one loin, shooting down to the front of the thigh or testes or vulva, frequency of micturition and vomiting, shivering, sweating, pallor, and partial collapse. These pains are followed by haematuria, containing blood and pus. The condition is RENAL COLIC.***

The treatment consists of two parts. One during an acute attack and the other during the interval.

Berberis vulgaris : there are radiating pains from the kidney to bladder. Pain from the kidney extends along the ureter or to liver, stomach, spleen, arresting breathing. Bubbling sensation in the region of the kidney. Frequent urination with the sensation as if some urine is left behind. Urine is thick mucus, and bright red, turbid, yellow or sandy.

Calcarea carb: irritable bladder, incontinence while walking, Urine is dark, brown sour, foul, or of strong odour. White urinary sediment with milky urine, at times bloody. Other constitutional characteristics are present.

Benzoic acid: there is insufficiency of the kidney, excess of uric acid, causing cystitis. Urine is hot dark brown, strong foul odour of horse urine. Bed wetting — sheets get stained brown. It has a uric acid diathesis. Pains suddenly change their locality.

Lithium carb: soreness of the bladder, pain is in the right kidney and the ureter. Pain in the bladder extends up to spermatic cord. Urine is scanty with much thirst, still the urine is scanty, turbid urine with mucus, scanty and dark acid sandy deposits.

Hydrangea: it is remedy for gravel, profuse deposits of white amorphous salts in the urine, therefore tendency to form stones. Urine is bloody and the drug acts on the ureters. It is claimed that Hydrangea arrests the formation of stones. Burning in uretha with frequent desire to urinate, difficult to start the urine. There is sharp pain in the loins.

Sarsaparilla: pain from the right kidney downwards. Urging to urinate before menses. There is severe pain at the conclusion of urination. Child screams before passing the urine; kidney colic and painful urination in children. Can pass urine only when standing and dribbles when sitting.

During the interval of the attacks, investigate the type of stones the patient is having, and find out the constitutional remedy which can be used during the period of lucid interval. One will see that the attacks become more mild and the stones pass out. The acidic urine shows two forms of stones. The commonest form is dark brown in colour, consists of calcium oxalate and gives rise to more acute symptoms. These have fine bristles with sharp pointed crystals, which cause bleeding and colour the calculus. Another form is of uric acid and urates mixed in varying proportions. These for light brown stones, round and branching, and are commonest stones in gouty subjects. Those who have high uric acid level usually deposit urates. Calculi are often multiple. In alkaline urine, phosphate stones are found.

There are certain drugs known to have action on these stones. In case of oxalate of lime Causticum, Kalisulph, Nat phos and Nitric acid have good effects. Benzoic acid, Ferrum met, Phosphoric acid, Ptelia, Stannum are known to have good effect and Urtica urens shows good effect on the urates.

Calcarea renalis: it is a urate of lime. There is great colic with intensity and passage of uric acid stones. This also useful in the tartar of the teeth and help resolve the formation of nodosity of stony hardness in the finger. But, all the same, a full history is necessary before one arrives at the right remedy. The patient needs to be educated on the importance of free fluid intake and to avoid those articles of daily food which are known to produce these stones.

4. ***Patient with peripheral oedema, mostly in the lower limbs, massive generalized anasarca for over some time, anorexia, diarrhoea, vomiting, and bouts of frequent attack of hypertension. It is probably NEPHROTIC SYNDROME.***

Nephrotic syndromes are common in children below 3 years where there is oedema over the face more marked. There is oliguria, while oedema is forming, massive proteinuria, urine becoming almost solid on boiling. Fatty casts, tubular cells, oval fat bodies are present.

Diet is very important. A high protein diet is advised. But salt should be restricted to 1gm/day. Fruits, fruit juices, eggs, bread, jam and honey may be given at breakfast. Fish and meat is permitted at lunch and dinner.

Arsenic alb: urine is scanty, burning, involuntary, bladder as if paralysed. Epithelial cells, cylindrical clots of fibrin, and globules of pus and blood. Feeling of weakness in abdomen after urination. Atony of the bladder causing paralysis and retention of urine. Urine is black as if mixed with dung.

Apis mel: burning and soreness when urinating. Dysuria causing last drop to scald, burn. Scanty high coloured urine,with casts, Albuminuria, with coffee ground sediment. Incontinence of urine at night but during day difficult, frequent and slow urination, must press to pass the urine. Stinging, burning pains while urinating.

Colchicum: more the discharge of urine more urging. Urine is hot , highly coloured, bloody and black almost like ink, black sediment.

Terebinthina: this is the remedy to be thought of when the urinary symptoms appear after exanthemata, and followed by violent bronchitis. Burning, drawing pain in the region of the kidney, along ureters, constant tenesmus, and strangury with bloody urine. Urine is smoky, with coffee ground, or thick, yellow and slimy sediment. Urethritis, nephritis. Scanty and suppressed urine.

Cantharis : constant desire to urinate. Intolerable tenesmus. Cutting before, during and after the urination. Urine burns, scalds with cutting pains, and intolerable urging. Urine is drop by drop.

5. ***Patient comes with sudden onset of fever, with rigors, malaise and pallor. Frequently nausea and vomiting. Pain and tenderness in the loins, and flanks, occasional haematuria, and frequency of urination every half an hour. It is ACUTE PYELONEPHRITIS.***

It is seen that whatever is the pathological picture, the expression of the patients do not alter very much. The drugs having action on the kidneys and bladder will be considered for pyelonephritis. Drugs like Apis, Berberis, Benzoic acid, Cantharis, Sarsaparilla, Lycopodium and Phosphorus can be considered. Signs and symptoms of these drugs have been mentioned under different diseases of the Urinary tract.

6. ***Patient complains of supra pubic-discomfort and pain, frequency of micturition, and there is discharge of pus at the end of the micturition or sometimes mixed with the urine. The condition is CYSTITIS.***

Cystitis can be of two forms: Acute cystitis and chronic cystitis. In acute cystitis at the onset, there is little amount of pus but in severe cases there will be haematuria also. The urine is ropy and with pus and mucus. Pain and tenderness in the hypogastrium. Micturition is frequent and painful.

In chronic cystitis, larger amount of pus and urine is alkaline, and contains ropy mucus. Pain is less severe, than in acute cystitis.

There are many causes to give cystitis-like residual urine, prostate enlargement, urethral strictures, stones of foreign bodies. Infection spreads to the bladder in most cases.

Apis and Cantharis are two important remedies the details about which are already mentioned earlier in connection with other inflammatory conditions of kidney.

Lachesis: characteristic symptom is sensation as if a ball is rolling in the bladder on turning over. The urine is almost black, frequent, foaming and dark. Has to urinate on lying down, day or night. Floating of black soot-like particles in the urine floating.

Lycopodium: the urging of urine is sudden and severe. Passage of urine was intense burning. There is sensation as if molten lead is passing through the urethra. Urine discharged is very scanty, turbid, dirty brownish red colour, and a peculiar smell of malt. Low potency of Lyco in 12 C is useful in repeated doses.

Pulsatilla: spasmodic pains in the bladder after urinating. Haematuria after urination. Urine dribbles when emotionally upset. Heavy pressure and cramp in the bladder after urination. Urging to urinate on lying on the back. Interrupted flow.

Clematis: tingling in urethra lasting for some time after urinating. Burning, frequent urination. Last drops cause violent burning. Urine starts and stops. Or dribble after urination. Difficult to evacuate the urine in one spell. There is mucus in the urine and not pus.

Equisetum: slight pain in the right kidney, then in the left. Urgent desire to urinate. Sharp pains at the root of the penis, at the close of urination. Retention and dysuria during pregnancy. Urine is cloudy, albuminuria. Has to get up many times at night to urinate.

7. ***Patient gives a history of pains, swelling, redness of the meatus, and scalding during micturition, also, usually in the morning, pus or muco-pus discharge. It is a case of URETHRITIS.***

Urethritis can be of two types — Specific, Gonococcal and non-specfic urethritis.

Cannabis sativa: itching and inflammatory swelling of the prepuce, glans and penis with deep redness and phimosis. Dragging and itching in the testes and tension in the spermatic cord when standing upright. Scanty burning urine passed drop by drop. Urine is turbid, white or reddish, as if mixed with blood and pus. Inflammation can be because of acute gonococcal infection, urethra is sensitive and has to walk with legs apart.

Cantharis: painful swelling of the genitals. Semen at times is bloody. Burning in urethra after sex. Strong desire and painful erection. Cutting burning pains from kidney down to urethra. Strangury, and can pass only few drops.

Petroselinum: tingling and lancinating pain in the urethra. Frequent but fruitless desire to urinate. Intense biting and pain deep in the urethra, milky fluid and albuminous yellow discharge from urethra. Often there is profuse pollutions in the morning.

Mercurius: glans penis and prepuce is swollen and testicles are swollen and hard. Frequent urging to urinate, and burning after urination. Greenish discharge from the urethra and urine is dark, scanty and bloody.

Medorrhinum: urethritis with heaviness in the prostate. Prostate is painful and enlarged with frequent and painful urination. Gleet, whole urethra is sore and painful. Profuse urination with craving for ice.

Thuja: there is inflammation of the prepuce and glans. Swelling of the prepuce. There is balanitis with warts on the prepuce. Offensive smelling genitals. Sweet smelling sweat on the genitals.

Argentum nit.: urine passes unconsciously day and night. Urethra is inflammed and painful, burning itching pain as from splinter. Emission of few drops after having finished. Divided stream. Early stage of gonorrhoea — profuse discharge and terrible cutting pain. Erection fails when sex is attempted. Impotency.

8. ***Patient complains that he finds it difficult to pass urine, but the bladder appears to be full on palpation and percussion. The condition is RETENTION OF URINE.***

Arnica: retention of urine in bladder from overexertion after labour. Bladder tenesmus with painful urination. The bladder feels sore and full. The pressure of urine hurts him, cutting pain in the kidneys. Involuntary dribbling with constant urging. Has to wait for a long time to commence urination. Urine has dark brick red sediment.

Arsenic alb: Retention of urine as if the bladder is paralyzed after childbirth. Atony of bladder in old persons. Urine is scanty and burning involuntary. Urine contains epithelial cells, cylindrical clots of fibrin, and globules of pus and blood, weakness feeling in the abdomen after urination.

Causticum: Paralysis of bladder after long retention of urine, and consequent incontinence. Involuntary passage of urine after coughing. Or any other condition causing intra-abdominal pressure. Retention of urine after labour or surgical operation. Burning in urethra after urinating and after sex. Insensibility of urethra while passing urine. Urine is black, cloudy white, itching of meatus.

Copaiva: Retention with pain in the bladder, anus and rectum. Burning pressure, painful urination by drops. Constant desire to urinate. Urine is acrid, scanty, bloody, odour of violets, greenish turbid colour, and urethra feels wide open.

Equisetum: Retention and dysuria during pregnancy, and after delivery. Sharp cutting and burning pain in the urethra while urinating.

Hyocyamus: Retention of urine after child-birth. Involuntary utination, bladder is paralyzed, no will to urinate. Frequent, scanty painful urination.

9. ***Patient complains that he has not passed urine for some time, but there is no evidence of distended bladder. Catheterization does not produce any result. The condition is SUPPRESSION OF URINE or ANURIA or OLIGURIA.***

Suppression may be due to obstruction of both the ureters, but kidney being healthy; tumour at the base of the bladder; Malformation of the ureters. This no passing of urine may be for days and there may be no symptoms. Thereafter he may turn restless, with contracted pupils, subnormal temperature, dry brown tongue, and muscular twitching. There may be vomiting in some cases. Death may result suddenly.

Suppression may be due to result of severe renal failure due to any acute or chronic causes. Acute nephritis, Sub-acute nephritis, Chronic pyelonephritis. Febrile state including heat-stroke. Here the high coloured urine passes, and may contain albumen casts. There may be urgent vomiting, diarrhoea and sweating.

Kali chloricum: Inflammation of the kidney causes urine to get suppressed. The urine is albuminous, scanty and supressed, has high phosphoric acid, with low total solids. Sometimes there is haematuria.

Opium: Loss of power of sensibility of bladder, paralytic atony of the bladder after laprotomy; retained, involuntary urination after fright.

Helleborus: Due to nephritis there is inflammation of the kidney and the urine may get suppressed, scanty, dark coloured, coffee ground sediment. Urine is retained although the bladder is over-distended during pregnancy, there is frequent urge to pass urine but very scanty discharge.

Solidago: It is a homeopathic replacement for a catheter. Dysuria with pain in the kidney. Kidneys are sensitive to pressure. Useful in chronic nephritis. Pain and tenderness in the kidney. Urine is dark red and brown, thick, and voided with difficulty.

Stramonium: Suppression of urine, specially during typhoid. The bladder is empty. Loss of power in the bladder in the aged. Stream flows slow. Rigor during urination.

In most of the cases the treatment is surgical and, therefore, surgeon should be consulted.

6 PEDIATRICS

- Concept of diseases & constitutions
- Deficiency diseases
- Attention — deficit disorders
- Rickets
- Scurvy
- Diphtheria
- Delayed Development
- Enuresis
- Teething
- Broncho-Pneumonia
- Diarrhoea
- Colics
- Febrile convulsions during teething
- Marasmus
- Kwashiorkor
- Infectious diseases
- Acute rheumatic fever
- Parotiditis
- Whooping Cough

Life seems to start when one male germ cell unites with female germ cell in the womb. They carry with them their traits, characters, and qualities — good and bad derived from their previous generations. The zygote so formed grows within the maternal environment where it is exposed to susceptibilities of the mother. From here on it grows to form a portrait. This is the beginning of the new code. As it grows within the influence of the maternal environment and the susceptibility modification of its traits, characters, and qualities start taking place. One will appreciate here how important it is to maintain the harmony of emotions, intellect and physical status of the mother. Gradually, as the zygote advances to further growth, it develops its own defense system in the form of Reticulo-endothelial system and the Psycho-Neuro Endocrine System. On any adverse or hostile influence on the environment in the womb it tries to modify itself in terms of emotional, intellectual and physical properties, and tries to remain in a balanced state. We call this a Constitutional State. Any hostile or adverse influence at this stage can throw this balanced system in an imbalance state or to what we call as a Diseased State.

Hahnemann meticulously studied these imbalanced cases and on the basis of their signs and symptoms grouped them into three classes (1) **Hypersensitive,** (2) **developing into defective metabolism or producing uncontrolled growth of tissue and** (3) **destructive tissue tendencies** to which he called ***Psoric, Sycotic and Syphilitic states* respectively.**

Many have tried to classify these constitutions of which Gruvagol's classification is practical.

Later Borland classified these constitutions into five groups of remedies on the basis of their characters:

1. Calcarea carbonica "Fair, Fat, Chilly and Lethargic" and includes Cal phos, Phosphorus, Silicea, Sanicula, Aethusa, Lycopodium, Causticum and Tuberculinum.

2. Baryta Carbonica, "Backward, delayed development " and includes Borax, Natrum Mur, Sepia, Aurum met, and Carbo vegetabilis.

3. Graphites" skin" and includes Capsicum, Psorinum, Antimonium crudum, and Petroleum.

4. Pulsatilla, "Warm blooded " and included Kali sulph, Sulphur, Thuja Bromium Iodum, Abrotanum and Fluoric Acidum.

5. Arsenic Alb " Nervy Type"and included, Chamomilla, Cina, Mag Carb, Ignatia, and Zincum.

The book on "Children Types" by Douglas Borland is well-known.

1. ***Child is showing progressive loss of subcutaneous fat, and is irritable and cries excessively, has sunken and lustureless eyes and sunken anterior fontanelle. Has lower body temperature, delayed milestones. This condition is MARASMUS.***

Marasmus is caused by insufficiency of diet, unsuitable feeding habits, disturbed mother-child relationship, inability to take food properly due to local lesions of the mouth, cleft palate, hare lip, thrush and chronic nasal obstruction. Lack of proper digestion due to chronic infection. Impaired absorption, defective metabolism or unsatisfactory utilization.

Education, and counselling is most important to the parents and people around. They should be taught and trained in avoiding and correcting the mentioned causes above. Protection against the infection and surgical correction of the defects. Treatment for stimulating the appetite shall be instituted. And to aid the digestion, enzyme preparations may be suggested.

Abrotanum: is a very powerful children's remedy in malnutrtion, failure to thrive, and marasmus. Child is very irritable, depressed, hyperactive, with a very negative behavior pattern. All of a sudden these changes and the mood is elevated. The Abrotanum disorders go to the intestine and when the mood is better there is better colon activity. This is seen with alternation of constipation and diarrhoea. In elders this is useful in conditions like Crohn's disease, colitis, irritable bowel syndrome. Another keynote is that the child has big appetite but lose weight. (Iod., Cina) and has no muscular strength.

Aethusa: it has inability to digest milk. There is marked aggravation of diarrhoea with warm milk. Improperly fed babies. There is so great weakness that they cannot hold their heads. This is often during the dentition time and summer time, the whole process sets in. There is brain fatigue, inability to think to fix attention. Restless, anxious and crying. There is attention deficit. Hungry after vomiting is the keynote.

Iodum: there is rapid metabolism causing rapid emaciation, weight loss. But the appetite is great. Better after eating, great debility, slightest efforts induce perspiration.

Silicea: helps defective nutrition, especially in children, due to defective assimilation. Scrofulous rickety children with large head and open fontanelles. Distended, hard and hot abdomen, wasted in legs and walking very slowly. Malnutrition and arrested development causing great emaciation.

Natrum muriaticum: emaciation is marked, due to defect in nourishment. They are particularly around the neck. They have ravenous appetite, and despite this grow thin. At least, they do not grow fat. This is similar to Iodine but the emaciation around the neck is characteristic of Natrum. It has well-marked thirst.

Magnesium carb: are puny and sickly from defective nutrition. There is severe diarrhoea that accompanies a cramping, much griping and rumbling in abdomen, with typically greenish stools. The child is poorly nourished, and the mouth is full of aphthous ulcers. These indications demonstrate poor nourishment.

2. ***A progressively losing weight child, in spite of much generalized oedema, cold extremities. Expression is apathetic but resents attention, wants to be left alone; watery offensive stools and dehydration, and with enlarged liver, a picture of malnutrition. The case is that of KWASHIORKOR .***

These cases need more than any therapeutic remedial measures, a proper care and management through adequate proteins. Prevention of early weaning, and education of mother. High protein and low fat, low sugar diet , palatable and digestible, with small and frequent feeds. There should be gradual increase in the diet. Vitamins A and B Complex, particularly Riboflavin, should be a part of the diet. Soyabean meals, maize flour, pulses and sweet banana, egg flip should be a part of the diet on recovery. Symptomatic treatment for the case as in marasmus, and, if there are any infections, they should be treated.

3. ***A child, usually between the age of four months and two years, restless and irritable, with sweating of head, and a large head compared to the body, beading of ribs, enlargement of epiphyses at wrist and with delay in dentition. The condition is RICKETS.***

This is a Calcium and Vit. D deficiency disorder. Apart from treatment here the supplementary diet rich in Vit. D and Calcium should be instituted.

Calciferol (Vit. D_2) is tasteless and can be added to milk. Fortified Milk with Vit. D_3 is advised. Fortified fish, oils should be added in later years of life.

Calcarea phos: especially called in for defective nutrition. Therefore useful in childhood as well in the puberty and old age. The child is thin and emaciated with sunken rather flabby abdomen, and predisposed to glandular and osseous diseases. The head is large, both the fontanelles are open, the cranial bones are unnaturally thin, and brittle. Late development of teeth, and has a curvature of the spine. Slow to learn to walk, and because of weak spine cannot support the body. The neck is so thin that it cannot support the head. Persistent vomiting of milk and suffers from colics. The stools are often green , slimy and lienteric, accompanied by flatus, and profuse. There is craving for ham or bacon; mentally very depressed, slow of comprehension. It is an excellent remedy to prevent rickets. If this fails, Silicea should be thought of.

Silicea: has typical characteristic features of rickets. The symptoms appear mostly from infancy, imperfectly nourished child, not from defective type of food it takes but from defective assimilation. Face and head have offensive sweat, slow learning to walk. The fibrous parts of the joint are swollen and inflamed, has a knob-like appearance. Silicea was found very useful in cases of after-effects of vaccination. Silicea is useful in scrofulous children where there are curvature of the bones, spinal as well lateral curvature and when there is caries of vertebral column.

Magnesia mur: is indicated in those with rickets where there is enlargement of the liver and when they are short in their growth. They are very easily susceptible to skin infection, particularly tinea ciliaris. There is sweat in the feet but not offensive as in Silicea.

Sulphur: often useful at the commencement of the disease, with a typical temperament. Sweats out the head, during sleep, and marked tendency to eruption on the skin. Because of the defective osseous growth the anterior fontanelle remain open too long. The child has a voracious appetite and greedily clutches whatever offered, as if it was starved. There is defective assimilation, and is not appropriated to the nourishment. So the child is always hungry and emaciated. The child looks shrivelled, and dried up, like little old man, the skin hangs in folds-wrinkled and flabby.

4. ***Child, usually between the age of 9 months to 2 years, complains of painful legs and is irritable. There is anaemia and characteristic subperiosteal haemorrhages in the ends of the long bones. The condition is SCURVY.***

Scurvy is a deficiency disorder found more common in artificially fed infants where thę plasma ascorbic acid is very low and vitamin C level is less than 0.1 (g.dl -l) in the leucocyte-platelet layer of the centrifuged blood — indicates deficiency. It is precipitated by febrile diseases, infections or diarrhoea.

The anaemia is usually hypochromic but occasionally a normochromic or megaloblastic anaemia is seen. Often this anaemia is due to iron deficiency — due to decreased absorption and loss due to haemorrhage. In the gums only if the teeth have erupted, common at the base of incisors. There will be swelling of gums with a thin purple line and fleshy mass. Scorbutic beading of the ribs due to backward displacement of sternum and costal cartilages. Low grade fever is common.

Carbo vegetabilis: acts upon the venous circulation, and capillaries blood seem to stagnate causing blueness, coldness and ecchymoses. Limbs are heavy and stiff and feel paralysed, want of muscular energy, paralytic weakness of the wrist, and of the fingers when holding anything, burning pains in the bones and limbs. Gums are retracted and bleed easily, painful while chewing. Bleeds when cleaning teeth.

Staphysagria: teeth turn black and have dark streaks through them, and cannot be kept clean.They crumble, decay on edges, scorbutic cachexia. In the mouth, there are pale bleeding gums, salivation and spongy gums bleed easily. Muscles of limbs feel very beaten and painful, joints are stiff.

More than selecting the remedies, most important is the diet. It is suggested to give orange juice to infants who are bottle-fed. And the nursing mothers should be encouraged to eat more of fruits and green vegetables and should be more careful about their diet. There should be supplement of ascorbic acid in the food to 1 g daily.

5. ***There is a complaint from the mother that child wets the bed often during night, or regularly. This condition is NOCTURNAL ENURESIS OR BEDWETTING.***

Nocturnal Enuresis or bedwetting, in common language, is an obstinate condition and needs a very close study of each case. It belongs to pseudo-psoric or tubercular miasm, and some cases belong to sycotic miasm.

Bed wetting by children beyond the age when control of urinary bladder should have been acquired due to delay in maturing physiological reflex bladder control.

Cina or santonin — active principle of Cina, and often indicated in wormy child. It is specially indicated when urine grows milky on standing. The general characters of Cina will be present — grinding of teeth, irritable temper and sour smell of the body. Hungry, and greater the hunger, greater the emaciation. The child sleeps on the belly or on the hands and knee.

Benzoic acid: urine is very hot, dark brown, strong foul smelling. Having odour of horses urine. Urine is ammonical in smell. The sheets on which the child sleeps get unusually stained brown.

Causticum: paralytic bladder from long retention of urine, and consequent incontinence. Involuntary urine during first sleep at night or from slightest excitement. Involuntary passage of urine on coughing or sneezing. Urine dribbles or passes slowly. And is passed better sitting. Urine is black, dark, cloudy white, and with itching of the meatus. Worse in winter and better in summer. Tendency to escape during the day on laughing or coughing or any extra exertion.

Sepia: like causticum, bedwetting is during the first sleep, or as soon as the child goes to sleep. Involuntary, worse coughing, sneezing, laughing, hearing sudden noise, fright or inattention. Urine stream is feeble, slow thick foul grity red adhesive sandy sediment — often bloody and milky.

Verbascum: bedwetting at night, worse on coughing. And the child has during the day constant dribbling. With the increase in pressure in bladder there is burning urination. It is found to be more useful in drop doses of mother tincture, in warm water three to four times a day. Verbascum oil is also used in some cases.

Equisetum: nocturnal bed wetting in children without any apparent cause except habit or with dreams or nightmares, when passing urine in bed. Otherwise there is constant desire to pass urine during the day. Frequent urination with severe pain at the close of urination. Use 30th potency.

Plantago: has considerable clinical reputation in the treatment of earache, toothache and bedwetting. There is tenderness over the kidney area, on pressure. Delayed and dribbling urine, and nocturnal bedwetting is due to laxity of sphincter. Irritable bladder that causes frequency of urination.

Rhus aromaticus: bedwetting is due to bladder atony, also for senile incontinence. There is severe pain during or at the beginning of urination. The urine is pale and albuminous. 10 drops of mother tincture a dose.

Apart from these remedial measures the patient should be advised to refrain from drinking water immediately before sleeping. Habit should be developed to pass urine before sleeping. At times excessive cold room or sleeping without the warm covering may cause this enuresis.

6. ***Child suddenly is seized with pain in the abdomen, becomes restless and cranky folds the legs near the abdomen and cries. This condition is COLIC.***

Children are often affected with severe abdominal pain called colic. There are many reasons those can be attributed to.

Many remedies can be thought of but the main remedies are :

Chamomilla: the child is whining, restless, spiteful, snappish, and want to be carried and held all the time. Complains are from anger and vexation. Distended abdomen, and spells of colic from time to time, flatulent colic after anger, with red cheeks. Griping in the region of umbilicus, and pain in small of the back, cutting wind colic more at night, worse urinating and better by warm application.

Cina: ill-humoured child, with bloated abdomen, twisting pain about about the navel, better on applying pressure.

Colocynth: agonizing cutting pain in abdomen causing patient to bend over double pressing on the abdomen, colicky pains are violent, cutting, griping, grasping, clutching or radiating. These pains come in waves, worse by least food or drink, during the colic the child lies on abdomen and screams.

Magnesia phos: severe griping colic, at time shooting upwards to stomach, better by hot application. Flatulent colic forcing the patient to bend double, relieved by rubbing, warmth, pressure accompanied with belching gas — that gives no relief. Bloated, full sensation in the abdomen, must loosen clothes, walk about and constantly pass flatus.

Nux vomica: colic is most common in nursing infants from stimulating food taken by mother. Flatulent distension with spasmodic colic, bowels gripe here and there, causing sore abdomen. Umbilical hernia of children due to constipation. Hiccough from over-eating, from cold or warm drink, sour taste in the mouth in the morning after eating. Nausea and vomiting with much retching. Nausea is better if patient can vomit. Spasms and over-sensitiveness and chilliness are three main points of Nux vom.

7. ***Mother informs that all these days the child was very good at studies and attentive but lately has started falling back in the class and cannot concentrate. It is a case of ATTENTION DEFICIT.***

Attention deficit child or learning disabled child is often very bright but have poor self-confidence, inadequate learning style or family history of abuse or neglect. There is absence of encouragement, or belief in themselves. They may be dyslexic, having auditory or visual problems. They do not have any inspiring role models. They may also have physiologic sequelae of their mother's drug or alcohol abuse in utero. This last cause may not be very pertinent in our Indian scenario. But some people who are pseudo-rich may indulge in these activities without knowing their consequences.

Nux vomica : children with extreme tension, they are hard driving with competitive spirit, and always strive to be number one. They tend to be irritable and perfectionist. Sensitive to light and noise, and have difficulty in sleeping. They wake up early in the morning at 3 a.m. and start thinking about the daily chore. They crave spices fatty food, and stimulants. Their physical problems are indigestion and constipation.

Chamomilla: these are angry children, and irritable to the extreme. Always complaining type — whine and cry.They reject whatever offered and do not seem to know what they want. Restless and want to be carried and rocked all the time. But they do not like to be touched. They tend to have intestinal colic and diarrhoea like chopped spinach.

Crotalus cascavella: these are fearful children and have characteristic fear of being alone. They always feel that someone is following them from behind : ghosts, spirits and snakes, they dream of hairy spiders, are talkative and hurried. They get into fits of rage, Hives usually in one part of body.

Natrum sulph: a medicine for depression developing after head injury. Depression primarily from being scorned in relationship situations. Child may feel very bad about himself, isolate himself and may even consider suicide. These children have tendency to experiment with drugs. On the physical side there may be warts or asthma.

Colocynthis: anger and indignation are the main feelings of these children. They are easily offended by insults, humiliation or feeling unappreciated. They are highly sensitive to pain.

Arsenic alb : very restless and insecure, with lot of anxiety about their health and often fear of death. Disproportionate terror of being left alone. Always worried about the germ contamination. These children are anxious like more adult like, than adults than their age. They are needy, whiny and impatient.

Bismuth subnitricum: children who cling desperately to the fingers of their parents. Just out of terror of being alone. Cannot remain alone for a moment not, even till the one comes out of the bathroom or toilet. Often very thirsty and has vomiting as soon the water reaches the stomach.

Hyoscyamus: act successively, silly jokes and show off, talk too much. They try to attract attention by whatever means. Throw tantrums. Jealousy is a problem. This can turn into malicious violence against the younger sibling. These children are precocious sexually and do masturbate in public. Bed wetting may be a persistent complaint.

Aethusa cyn: one very characteristic symptom here is inability to think or fix attention. Usually happens to students who overwork beyond their capacity. And then there is inability to think and fix attention. They become restless and anxious and irritable. The results is seen at failure in the examination. These children are idiotic looking, and are awkward in their behaviour.

Baryta carb: this brings help to scrofulous children who are backward — mentally and physically. Dull and apathetic, do not grow and develop. They are shy of strangers, forgetful, have loss of memory, mental weakness, are irresolute and have lost confidence in themselves. Are bashful and timid. Mental grasp is very slow. Deficient memory. Cannot remember and learn.

Carcinocin: there is a great fear of failure. Fear in examination, fear of heights and crowd. Difficult concentration. There is Autism and mental retardation. Hyperactivity. Hyperactivity with a result, cannot fix attention. Attention-deficit syndrome, has obsessive compulsive disorder.

Medorrhinum: they are desperate, sad, tearful and fearful individuals. People with weak memory and cannot concentrate. Suddenly loses the thread in conversation. Forgets name, errands, repeats again and again. Apprehensive and anticipates events. Many cases of stunted growth and arrested development in children are due to latent gonorrhoea.

Lyssin (rabies nosode): this suits children who have been sexually abused. These are the most violent and difficult to handle. There is often a history of dog bite or is scared of dogs, fear of water, claustrophobic. These children may aggravate by sound or sight of running water and bedwetting may be a problem. There is torment followed by rage.

Scorpion androcotonos amurreuxi helbraeu (Tincture of the living animal): children who lack conscience and compassion for the suffering of others. These children can be extremely violent, hurting may even commit murder. Parents of these children often fear that these children are heading for life of criminal violence. They are detached from other people and like to remain alone. These children view the world from a small hole in the rocks like a scorpio does. They are self-centered, indifferent to pleasure or pain and live in a self-imposed isolation.

Bufo rana (Toad): this is a medicine for slow, coarse children, with particularly strong interest in sex and masturbation. They do not comprehend well, have dull look , thick lips. They rely on the basic instincts and instant gratification. Music and bright objects are intolerable. They are averse to being misunderstood. Seizures are common.

Zincum metallicum: the children here are fidgety and restless. Their nervous system is hyperactive with twitching, jerking, and even convulsions. Restless legs in bed is characteristic. Sensitive, complaining type. They are dull and make lots of mistakes in speaking and writing.

Baryta carb: dependence is the main character, for anything that he is supposed to do on his own needs a help. They are passive and indecisive. Delayed development academically and socially. They find it difficult to grasp concepts or skills. They hide behind their mothers, and are timid about trying anything new. Prone to chronic tonsillitis, with huge tonsils. Crave eggs.

We are observing that more and more children are being labelled as Autistic or Attention-deficit. And if we study these emotional phases in their life one can possibly restore them to normalcy.

8. ***Ten month child brought with the complaint of no teething yet, but instead many constitutional disturbances like fever, convulsions and diarrhoea from time to time. This is a case of DELAYED TEETHING.***

We are often confronted with children of a very tender age with the problem of dentition. Cutting of tooth is truly a physiologic process and the healthy children pass of that period without any complaint or any constitutional signs and symptoms. No doubt there is increased activity during that period of dentition and if there are predisposition to any disorder the eruption of teeth will occur with much pain and suffering, accompanied with constitutional disturbances, often of a marked degree, such as diarrhoea, dysentery, spasms, convulsions, febrile states, abscesses in the middle ear, disturbances of digestion, meningeal congestions and inflammations.

Thrush and stomatitis are of psoric origin, but when we see a true ulcer in the mouth or in any other adjoining mucous surface, it is no more a Psoric. The true ulcer is syphilitic, or tubercular in origin. Any glandular involvement — swellings or induration taking place in the teeth or the dental arch are of syphilitic or of tubercular diathesis. When we come across haemorrhage in the mouth, excessive bleeding of the gums or if they are soft we attribute that to tubercular diathesis. Gums bleed at the slightest touch, gums recede from the teeth or they are soft and spongy and bleed while brushing. The dental arch is imperfect, often decaying, or becoming carious before they are entirely through the gums, or before they are perfectly developed.

Calcarea carb: has tardy teething and late walking. They do not want to put their feet on the ground, are emaciated, with big head and belly. These children are susceptible to cold, and take cold easily in the chest. Dull and lethargic — do not want to play. They sweat profusely with a sour smell to the perspiration. Offensive taste to the mouth, with bleeding gums.

Calcarea phos: affects the nutrition of the bones and glands. There is slow development of the teeth, slow in walking, neck is too thin to hold the head. On examination we may find adenoids growing. As there is delayed teething, there is decaying of the teeth after they erupt. Often there is convulsion without fever.

Silicea: in children there is defective nutrition due to imperfect assimilation. Teeth crumble, break down, lose their enamel, become rough and carious, abscesses at the root of the teeth; they are sensitive to cold. Gums have painful boils on them.

Kreosotum: very rapid decay of the teeth with spongy and bleeding gums, teeth are dark and crumbly, black spots on the teeth, putrid odour of the mouth, has a very painful dentition.

Mercurius vivus: there is increased saliva flow during sleep. Gums are spongy, recede and bleed easily. Teeth are hollow, black, pain is worse on heat and cold.

9. ***An infant in the process of teething develops fever which rises suddenly causing the infant to go into convulsion, the case is FEBRILE CONVULSION DURING TEETHING.***

Belladonna: as already stated earlier, ailments from dentition can be produced in susceptible individuals which may include fever and convulsions. These are plethoric children with red face, bilious children and lymphatic temperament who are very jovial and intelligent otherwise but violent when sick. It acts on nerve centers producing twitching, convulsions and pain. It produces an active congestion. Violence and suddenness of attack are the characteristic. Pupils are dilated and staring and brilliant. Eyes snap, and move quickly.

Chamomilla: it is hypersensitive to pain. Irritable and colicky baby. Mostly during their teething period. Always better from being carried, warm and wet weather, worse from anger and at night. Swelling or redness of cheek, one cheek red and hot and the other cold and pale. Child is chilly yet gets easily overheated. Thirst during fever.

Helleborus: this remedy is for low state of vitality, and serious diseases. There is general muscular weakness. The child is dull, stupid-looking, slow of perception or apathetic, slow in answering. Picks at lips and clothes. And has sinking sensation.

It is advisable to give a tepid water sponging and keep cologne water strips on the forehead and abdomen; keep the room airy and cool.

10. ***Mother of the teething child complains that the child has started suddenly loose watery stools of variable colour and consistency. TEETHING DIARRHOEA.***

In fact there is no condition like teething diarrhoea but it is a diarrhoea during the teething process in some predisposed or susceptible children, this constitutional complaint is given importance in Homoeopathy.

Calcarea carb: children crave for eggs, and eat dirt, and other indigestible things and are prone to diarrhoea. During teething there are many complaints, and are susceptible to cold. Sweats easy and has a sour sweat. The stools are chalky, gray or green, watery stools, the stools are first hard then pasty and then liquid. Worsens on eating and drinking. Undigested stools. This associated with difficult and delayed dentition.

Aethusa Cynapium: this remedy is suited to infants, teething children, having cholera disorders and the elderly. It has undigested, thin, greenish stool preceded by colic with tenesmus followed by exhaustion and weakness. There is intolerance of milk, vomits everything taken.

Borax: it is suited to children during the period of dentition. To children with lax skin and muscles getting cold in cold and wet weather. Colic with tendency to diarrhoea after every feed or a meal. Burning in the rectum after stool, and stools turning green or persistently green like boiled starch, or loose pasty offensive stools. There are bleeding gums and painful gum boils.

Chamomilla: diarrhoea during dentition, from cold or from anger. Stools are hot, green, watery, fetid slimy with colic. Stools can be sour, grass green, slimy. Yellow-green or lienteric, smelling like bad egg. And look like chopped eggs and spinach. Develops haemorrhoids with fissures. The child is spiteful and uncivil. Irritable.

Ferrum met.: pain in the teeth relieved by icy cold water, but stomach won't tolerate any food and causes distension. Diarrhoea is painless, worse while eating. Stools are undigested. Useful in summer diarrhoea.

Ipecacuhana: it has persistent nausea and vomiting. Dysenteric stools with tenesmus while straining. Stools brown, grass or yellow green, frothy molasses-like or slimy. Or pitch-like green as grass, with griping at the navel. At times there are lumps of mucus in the stool.

Podophyllum: it is remedy for bilious constitution. Headache alternating with diarrhoea. It is of a long-standing nature, early in the morning with the teething process, with hot glowing cheeks. Gurgling through the bowels, profuse putrid stools gush out painlessly. Green water, fetid and profuse, followed by weakness. Summer diarrhoea. The stools are involuntary in sleep, when passing flatus. Constipation alternating with diarrhoea. Often there is prolapse of rectum.

Rheum palmatum: the grand key note of this remedy is sourness. The stools are sour, the taste is sour and the whole body is sour. No amount of washing helps. Such a condition is peculiar to children during the dentition, or in nursing children. Shivering with stool is characteristic. The colic is severe, compelling one to bend double.

11. ***Usually a child between the age of 5-15 years. Patient comes with a sudden fever, fleeting joint pains, affecting large joints, which are swollen red and tender, malaise and loss of appetite. This condition is probably ACUTE RHEUMATIC FEVER.***

On examination we may find heart murmurs, new or changed murmurs if there has been a history earlier of similar episode. There may be transient diastolic murmur due to mitral valvulitis. The arthritis associated with rheumatic fever is classically fleeting in type, affecting knees, elbows and ankles. As the inflammation in one joint recedes, another becomes affected. ECG may show signs of pericarditis (raised ST segment) or myocarditis (inverted or flattened T wave) or may show some cardiac arrhythmia.

The rest shall be for at least 4-6 weeks till the intensity of the murmur is reduced, or has become stabilized. and the sleeping pulse rate is below 100/pm. The convalescence may take at times more than 6 months. Throat swabs are cultured for Group A Streptococcus, ESR and C-reactive proteins are elevated.

If there are symptoms of throat it is necessary to treat them first to avoid further infection.

Belladonna: there is sore throat with red fauces and pain causing irritation, dry tickling cough, short and mostly at night. Stitches in the chest while coughing. Larynx is very painful. Throat is dry and hot. Throbbing all over. Throbbing in the carotids and temporal artery. Palpitation from least exertion, rapid but weakened pulse, at times the pulse is full hard and tense. Joints are swollen, red shining with red streaks radiating. Pains are shifting.

Aurum met: sore throat of Aurum is peculiar, stitching when swallowing pain in glands. Tonsils are swollen are ulcerated. Boring and burning pains are predominate. The pulse is rapid, feeble and irregular. Sensation as if heart stopped beating. Oppression of the heart.

Mercurius: sore throat, smarting and burning, difficult swallowing, with typical attack like tonsillitis. Palpitation in the heart on slight exertion. Awakes with the cardiac tremor. Pulse is irregular, quick, strong intermittent.

Rhus tox: soreness in the throat, better on warm drinks. Pains in joints are tearing, shooting and stitching and the joints feel bruised and stiff. This develops more in cold damp weather. The onset may start after an attack of Influenza. Rheumatic pains spread over a large surface.

Kalmia: affects the nerves, heart and circulation and a rheumatic remedy. Heart's action is tumultuous, rapid and visible. Fluttering of heart with anxiety. Pains are sharp burning shooting, radiating to the left scapula and arm. Palpitation is worse on leaning forward.

Spigelia: violent, audible palpitation, throbbing of carotids, subclavian arteries, radiating to throat, arms and scapular soreness, purring in the region of the heart. Pulse is intermittent with palpitation weak.

Recurrences are almost common when persistent cardiac damage is present. And appropriate medicine should continue.

12. ***Child essentially looks toxic, and the condition gradually worsens with low grade fever and tachycardia. The disease is local, its manifestations are a membrane that is developing in the throat. This is caused by Corynebacteria diphtheriae, a gram-positive club shaped bacillus. The condition is DIPHTHERIA.***

There are four varieties of Diphtheria:

1. **Nasal Diphtheria**, is characterized by presence of a unilateral, sero-sanguinous nasal discharge that crusts around the external nares.

2. **Pharyngeal diphtheria** is associated with the greatest toxicity and is characterized by marked tonsillar and pharyngeal inflammation. A tough grayish white membrane that is formed by fibrin, bacteria, epithelial cells, mononuclear cells and polymorphs, firmly adherent to the underlying tissue. Regional lymphadenopathy is prominent and produces the so-called bull neck.

3. **Laryngeal diphtheria** is extension of the membrane from the pharynx. It may produce acute circulatory failure around 10th day. Some neurological manifestations may occur early in disease. Palatal or pharyngeal wall paralysis may occur. Or several weeks after its onset cranial nerve palsies, peripheral neuropathy may develop.

4. **Cutaneous diphtheria** is seen with cases of burns and people with poor hygiene. Constitutional symptoms are uncommon.

In nasal diphtheria there is an anterior nasal discharge, often blood stained with excoriation of the nostrils and upper lip. Nasal obstruction is present but without any constitutional symptoms or very few symptoms and this condition continues for weeks before any active advice is sought. A grayish-white membrane is seen on the septum and the inferior turbinate. Diphtheria bacillus are found in the membrane.

Kali bichrom: useful in the early stages of the disease. Fullness at the root of the nose. Sinusitis with distress. Loss of smell. Nasal discharge is thick, ropy, greenish. Tough elastic plugs, and large clinkers. Post-nasal drip of thick mucus. Coryza with obstruction of the nose. There is ulceration of the nasal septum, fetid smell because of retention of this discharge. These symptoms call for its use in nasal diphtheria.

Mercurius cyanatus: it affects most prominently mouth, throat, and larynx. These symptoms associated with prostration, coldness and cyanosis are leading indications, which indicate its use in diphtheria. There is necrotic destruction of soft parts of the palate and fauces. Intense redness of the fauces, swallowing is very difficult. Much thick grayish membrane in the throat. Use 30 c potency.

Nitric acid: the nose is red and has a scurfy tip, nose bleed is dark, clotted with chest affection. Chronic nasal catarrh, with yellow offensive corrosive discharge, sneezing frequent, without coryza, during sleep. There is coryza with sore and bleeding nostrils. These symptoms indicate nasal diphtheria.

Faucial diphtheria is now not as common as it used to be in the past but in developing countries like ours it is still seen in practice. The onset is gradual with general listlessness, pallor and often headache, and vomiting, there is low grade temperature, sore throat and dysphagia. Initially the throat is just congested but soon there is characteristic creamy white patch situated on the congested surface. Slowly these patches spread beyond tonsils, to fauces, soft palate uvula, and pharyngeal wall. If this progresses beyond second week, myocardial damage and failure may occur.

Kali bichrom and mercurius cyanatum are again indicated with their characteristic symptoms.

Bromium: the disease begins in the larynx and runs up croup with the croupy sound, there is much rattling in larynx, with breathing and while coughing. But there is no choking.

Carbolic acid: glazed ulcerated patches inside the lips and cheeks. Burning in the mouth to stomach. Fauces are red and covered with exudation. Uvula threatened and shrivelled. Putrid discharge. Fetid breath, The face is dusky red, white about mouth and nose.

Lachesis: aphthous and denuded spots, with burning and rawness, gums are bluish, swollen, spongy, and easily bleeding. Tongue is swollen, burns and cracked at the tip. Empty swallowing is agonizing, liquids are swallowed with less pain and solids with least pain. Fetid breath and the prostration is out of proportion to the appearance of the throat.

Diphtherinum: trituration of the diphtheric membrane to the point of 6c and dilutions are made from the diphtheric toxin. Diphtherinum is useful as a prophylactic in Diphtheria and post-diphtheria complications. Like paralysis, or when antidiphtheria vaccination is used. The indications are chiefly clinical — the fluctuating temperature, very little pain membrane in vertical folds, on posterior wall of the throat, when the membrane first appeared. Dark red swelling of the tonsils, and palatine arches.

13. ***Usually a child reports with fever, malaise, headache, and anorexia. And associated pain over the parotid glands with sore throat and stiffness of the neck. The condition is ACUTE EPIDEMIC PAROTIDITIS or MUMPS.***

The prodromal symptoms are non-specific and pain that develops over the parotids may be either unilateral or bilateral. This infection is spread by droplet infection. Central nervous system involvement is the commonest as extra-salivary gland manifestation of mumps. One-third of the patients develop epididymo-orchitis, they develop mumps after puberty. And bilateral testicular involvement results in sterility in a small percentage of patients. Myocarditis, mastitis, oophoritis and polyarthritis may also occur.

Treatment is symptomatic but attention should be given to adequate nutrition and mouth care.

Belladonna: high fever with hot head and cold limbs. No thirst with fever. There is great sensitiveness, particularly of special senses, sensitive to light, to slightest noise, or even if someone touches the bed. There is congestion in the throat, worse on the right side. The throat feels constricted. There is swelling and redness on the parotid gland.

Mercurius proto iod: Mercurius iodatus flavus: it has strong affinity for glands. The cervical and parotid glands are enormously swollen, and characteristic coating of the tongue. Much accumulation of tenacious mucus in the throat. Sensation of lump and constant inclination to swallow. This is a right-sided remedy.

Lycopodium: this is again a right-sided remedy. With swelling and suppuration of tonsils. Painful deglutition, worse by cold drinks.

Mercurius Bin Iod: Mercurius iodat. Ruber.: The affection of the inflammation of the lymphatic glands is mostly on the left side. The fauces are dark red. Stiffness of muscles of throat and neck.

Lachesis: the throat is livid, purple sore throat that begins on the left side, sore throat worse on the left side. The pain is aggravated by hot drinks, worse swallowing the saliva.

Kali bichrom: the parotid glands are swollen, with relaxed and oedematous uvula pseudo-membranous deposits on the tonsils. The mucus in the throat is very sticky. All the signs and symptoms are indirect evidences of mumps. A trained physician can easily locate the correct remedy.

Bromium: has enlarged parotids and goiter. Left-sided mumps. The glands are hard but seldom suppurate. Chief complications are orchitis and much less often oophoritis. Orchitis is rare before puberty. But in young adults who are sexually active it is frequently noticed. This complication develops about 10 days after the acute attack of mumps has subsided. It starts with sudden pyrexia with one of the testes getting enlarged and tender. This inflammation settles down in a week or ten days. Sub-fertility is common when both the testes are involved and anxiety of this can cause impotency of psychogenic origin.

Clematis erecta: Orchitis with heavy, hanging, or retracted testes. Induration with bruised feeling in the testes. Usually the right testes is affected. There is swelling of the spermatic cord with burning and soreness. Burning in penis during emission of semen during sex.

Pulsatilla nigricans: orchitis from sitting on cold floors. Pain from abdomen to testicles. Burning down left spermatic cord. Epididymitis. Testicles hang down. Bloody emissions. This is often associated with gonorrhoea.

Staphysagria: slow development of atrophy of the testicles after mumps. In females there is ovarian pain going into the thighs, worse by pressure. Also keep a close watch on the general characteristics of the drug.

There are neurological complications but they pass off quickly. Symptomatic treatment should be instituted.

14. ***A child with running nose and watering of the eyes, with malaise and temperature develops short dry cough, which turns persistent, and individual cough becomes grouped together. Probably it is a case of WHOOPING COUGH.***

This is a disease of the childhood, with 90% cases occurring below the age of 5. During the catarrhal stage the patient is highly infectious, malaise, anorexia, mucoid rhinorrhoea, and conjunctivitis is present. The paroxysmal stage has characteristic paroxysms of cough and classic whoop is seen only in younger children. And these paroxysms usually end in vomiting. This stage lasts for about two weeks, and may be associated with several complications, like bronchitis, lobar pneumonia, atelectasis, rectal prolapse and inguinal-hernia.

If the disease is recognized in the catarrhal stage then treat according to the symptoms. The most common remedies that resemble at this stage are **Allium cepa, Euphrasia, Arum triphyllum, Hepar sulph** etc. (**The details can be seen under respiratory chapter**).

In the paroxysmal stage the most important remedies like **Drosera, Corallium rub., Mephitis, Antimonium tart** and **Ipecac** are often indicated.

Drosera rotundifolia: it affects markedly the respiratory organs. Spasmodic cough, which resembles typical whooping cough. The characteristic cough is mostly aggravated in the evening and at midnight. And the patient holds his sides for relief. Everytime there is a spell of cough it ends into glairy mucus being brought out. He is better in open air, and worse after measles, singing, laughing, stooping. Worse on talking and taking cold food.

Corallium rubrum: used in Whooping cough where the attack comes with rapid coughs followed by exhaustion. Air passages feel cold on deep inspiration. The cough is dry, spasmodic, reverberating machine-gun cough, and at times profuse secretion dropping through posterior sinuses. After continuous cough, mucus is brought out.

Mephitis putorius: spasmodic cough or whooping cough. Few paroxysms in the day but many at night. Cough is violent, suffocative, spasmodic, nervous and worse on talking or drinking.

Pertussin: this drug can be used even as a preventive, for whooping cough and to treat the disease. Spasmodic cough during influenza when not related to whooping cough can be used.

Cuprum met: cough in violent paroxysm but better by cold drink. Whooping cough is better by swallowing water after the vomit, and the spasm with purple face. Audible sound of drinking.

There are respiratory diseases which may please be referred to at **Respiratory chapter** — like Pneumonia and asthma.

15. ***Child passes stools that are offensive, yellow in the beginning, then greenish slimy and mixed with curds of undigested food, Vomiting may or may not be present. The condition is ACUTE CATARRHAL OR DYSPEPTIC DIARRHOEA.***

16. ***Child passes greenish stools, slimy and often contains mucus, streaks of blood; fever and abdominal distention, with tenderness on pressure over the region of colon. The condition is INFANTILE INFLAMMATORY DIARRHOEA or ENTEROCOLITIS.***

17. ***Child has watery stools, foul smelling, green, and containing mucus, the stools turn gradually paler; acute abdominal pain with fever, prostration and collapse. EPIDEMIC DIARRHOEA.***

All these diarrhoea are collectively termed INFANTILE DIARRHOEA since they are common in childhood and infancy.

These children quickly go into dehydration and it must be combated on war footing. There are two ways that one can take — through ORS(Oral rehydration solution) and intravenous rehydration.

For correction of mild or moderate dehydration is best carried out by giving a glucose-electrolyte solution. There are many such commercially available solutions in the market But the WHO recommendation is Sodium 90; Potassium 20; Chloride 80; Bicarbonate 30; and glucose 111; mmol.L -1. Composition of ORS by weight should be Sodium chloride 3.5 grams, Sodium bicarbonate 2.5 grams, Potassium chloride 1.5 grams, and glucose anhydrous 20 grams per litre of ORS solution.

If this ORS is not readily available, Sugar Salt Solution (SSS) can be effectively used.

In 200 ml of clean drinking water add 2 finger pinch of salt. Stir the mixture with a clean spoon till the salt is fully dissolved. The solution should taste just salty. Next add a spoonful of sugar (jaggery). Stir this mixture till the sugar fully dissolves. Give this mixture to the child after every stool or sip by sip if there is vomiting along with the loose stools.

Intravenous rehydration is required only for severely dehydrated individuals with features of collapse — Sodium chloride 4.0 g., Sodium acetate 6.5 g., Potassium chloride 1.0 g. and glucose 9.0 g per liter. These diarrhoea treatment solutions are readily available in bottles. Several of these bottles are required to overcome the dehydration.

Arsenic alb: ill-effects of food poisoning, eating ice, poor diet, watery fruits, sea bathing and travelling are main causes. It affects the entire digestive tract, the lips are dry, parched, and cracked — the patient often licks them, patient is better always by warm drinks. Fruits in general cause stomach to get irritated. Burning pains in the rectum; useful in cholera; small offensive dark stool with much prostration.

Podophyllum: gastroenteritis is the characteristic complaint With colicky pains and bilious vomiting. Stools are watery and jelly like mucus, painless and profuse, gushing and offensive.

Veratrum album: diarrhoea is very painful, watery, copious. This is followed by great prostration and forcibly evacuated stool. When vomiting accompanies veratrum is more indicated.

Jalapa: it is a powerful purgative and hence affects intestines and stomach. It causes and cures colic and diarrhoea. The child is quiet all through the day but screams and tosses about all night. Colic, stools watery, muddy or sour, with general coldness and blueness of face.

Magnesia carb: milk passes undigested, in nursing children, preceded by griping, colicky pain. Stools are frothy, greenish like scum on the frog's pond. Sour stool with tenesmus. Belching sour, and vomiting of bitter water.

Rheum palmatum: it is for nursing infants and children, during dentition and suited to pregnant and nursing women. The whole child smells sour, even washing does not remove it. Mostly during difficult dentition. The stools are pappy, sour, brown, green, fermented and slimy, worse in the evening.

Chamomilla: the stools are hot, green, watery, foetid, slimy with colic. Chopped white and yellow mucus, like chopped egg and spinach. Mostly during dentition and the child is very irritable and snappy.

18. *Mother complains that the child often has abdominal pains, capricious or ravenous hunger, associated with loss of weight, irregular bowels, and at times diarrhoea, grinding of teeth at enuresis. The child is suffering from WORMS INFESTATION.*

There are many types of worms that infest the intestines collectively known as helminthiasis, and have variable signs and symptoms. The most common are ascarides lumbricoidis, oxyuris vermicularis, and hookworms, tapeworms, taenia saginata.

The symptoms can be from simple headache, constipation, nocturnal enuresis, irritability, itching in the rectum, to more severe complaints of convulsions.

Cina artemisia: it contains an alkaloid santonin. There is irritation of nose, causing constant desire to rub, pick or press into it. Grinding of teeth at night during sleep. Restless sleep and nocturnal enuresis. The worms are mostly roundworms and pin-worms. The child tosses about and restless during dentition, twitching spasms due to worms. They are hungry all the time but emaciate. The child lies on belly or on hands and knees in sleep.

Teucrium marum: has strong symptoms of worms infestation, irritation of anus and nose. More of threadworm infestation. The child is oversensitive and has a desire to stretch, has chronic nasal catarrh with atrophy with large offensive crusts. Nasal polyp ozaena and loss of sense of smell.

Filix mass: It is a male fern and is recognized as a vermifuge. There is bloating, gnawing and boring in bowels, worse on eating after sweet things, diarrhoea and vomiting. Itching of the nose, pale face with blue rings around the eyes. There is ineffectual urging to stool — pappy stools. Often there is constipation. Tincture of the fresh root or grated root maceration is used. This is primary remedy for expelling tapeworms.

Ferrum met: Vomiting after eating is a keynote and mostly after midnight. Diarrhoea while eating, nightly spluttering of undigested food. And spits up food by mouthful and vomiting without nausea. There is heat and burning in the stomach. Itching at the anus due to ascarides or worms in children.

Sabadilla: There is constipation, itching and crawling in the anus, alternating with itching in the nose or ears. Stools are burning, frothy, loose brown, which floats on the water. Pinworms crawling in the rectum and anus. There is multiple worm infestation. There are more reflex symptoms of worms with twitching, convulsive trembling.

Chenopodium anthelminthica: Oil of chenopodium has been used for hookworm or roundworm. The most characteristic pain of chinopodium is dull pain below the angle of the right scapula nearer the spine than that of Chelidonium. Oil is used in 10 minim doses every 2 hours; three such doses for hookworm.

19. ***Patient is brought with intense malaise, fever, rigors, severe headache, photophobia and vomiting. Often irritable and likes to lie down still, there is stiffness of the neck but consciousness is not impaired, but often is delirious. The condition is MENINGITIS.***

Meningitis is an emergency that has a high mortality even in countries where the health care system is well-developed. Viral meningitis is a self-limiting condition. Untreated bacterial meningitis is lethal. Immediate treatment should be started.

Acute simple meningitis is most often in tubercular or scrofulous children. This simple form is most common in the first two years of life and arises idiopathically or from injuries to the head. This is also accompaniment, or sequel, to the acute exanthemata, and occurs in connection with the diseases of the ear.

Aconite: a typical aconite picture of anxiety and violence is present. The skin is hot and dry and child tosses about and rolls, not keeping still. Screams as it pains. Flushed face and injected eyes, dry, burning heat with high fever.If these features are not relieved promptly one should think of Ferrum phos.

Ferrum phos.: throbbing headache with sensitive scalp. Headache is better by cold application. First stages of fever of unknown origin. It now stands between activity of Belladonna and Aconite.

Belladonna: sun-stroke and Meningitis are two main causes of the headaches and fever. Throbbing and hammering headaches, worse on the temples. There is no thirst with fever. Headaches with brilliant eyes and wide dilated pupils. Feet are icy cold. Perspiration dry only on the forehead.

Gelsemium: great prostration and headache. Chill with aching and languor. Chills up and down the spine, with cold hands and feet. Thirst is absent. Headaches are accompanied by blurring of sight and relieved by passing copious urine.

Helleborus niger : the action of Helleborus n. causes actual inflammatory states of the brain and meninges. Drowsiness is leading keynote of meningitis in Helliborus. Such condition is found when effusion has taken place from the inflamed membranes. The forehead is wrinkled, there are automatic movements of one arm and one leg while the other is paralyzed, the head rolls from side to side, with screams; drinking water greedily, chewing motion of jaws, urine is scanty or entirely suppressed. Limbs are cold, chill with fever sweat and aversion to cover.

20. *There is sudden onset of headache and drowsiness, with fever with stupor or convulsive seizure. The condition is VIRAL ENCEPHALITIS.*

In far east countries like India we have frequent epidemics of this Japanese B arbovirus. It causes very severe form of encephalitis with high mortality rate.

In Indian situation, when the epidemics of encephalitis raged in Assam, Andhra, Eastern Bengal, three remedies were outstanding in action — Belladonna, Apis, and Gelsemium. During these epidemics Central Council for Research in Homoeopathy had worked in these areas and provided their expertise in this field with very significant results.

21. *After a week or so of malaise, the child develops fever, signs of meningeal irritation, drowsiness, squints — one should suspect TUBERCULOUS MENINGITIS. History of tuberculosis or exposure to tuberculous infection should confirm the diagnosis.*

The early symptoms are very insidious. A slight irregular fever with constipation and occasional vomiting is common. Occasionally pain and discomfort in the neck may also be present. There is diminution or exaggeration of tendon reflexes. The irritative stage of fever, headache, neck rigidity, vomiting, photophobia occurs. There is alteration in the size of the pupils.

The patient after this diagnosis, should preferably be transferred to the hospital.

Apis mellifica : Apis produces serous inflammation with effusion membranes of the brain. There is swelling and puffing up of various parts, edema with red rosy hue, stinging pains, soreness and intolerance of heat, and from slightest touch.

Sudden shrill cry is characteristic in Meningitis and Hydrocephalus.

22. *Patient has cough, with frothy expectoration developing gradually after fever and "cold", followed by bronchitis, general malaise, a cough that produces shortness of breath. This is probably ACUTE BRONCHOPNEUMONIA.*

Bronchopneumonia is much more common in winter. In infants and small children these cases fall in two groups: *Primary* — The infecting agent usually is pneumococcus which causes a sudden rise of temperature, 104 ° F- 105 ° F, often with vomiting and convulsion. The child looks sick, the ribs are sucked in during respiration, flapping of alae nasi and the signs of consolidation are more clear to elicit. *Secondary* Broncho-pneumonia arises as a complication of measles, whooping cough, or of debilitating conditions as marasmus and streatorrhoea.

Antimonium tartaricum: it affects the mucous membranes, specially of the bronchial, and lungs. The therapeutic application is confined largely to the respiratory diseases. Rattling of mucus with little expectoration has been the guiding symptom. The respiration gets impeded due to great accumulation of mucus with coarse rattling. The child wants to be carried erect, and clings to the attendants. They cannot suck at the nipple and go out of breath. The cough is excited by eating, with pain in chest. The chest seems full but little raised.

Ipecacuanha: there is dyspnoea and constant constriction in the chest. Incessant cough, violent with every breath, continued sneezing and coryza with wheezing cough, bubbling rales, loose coarse rattling in the chest without expectoration. The child becomes stiff and blue in the face.

Grindelia robusta: indicated in chronic bronchial cough, when attended with profuse tenacious expectoration that gives relief. Breath stops when falling asleep and starts with waking up, gasping for breath.

Kali carb: dry cough about 3 a.m. with stitching pains. Asthmatic wheezing, worse by least motion. Swallows the expectoration, copious and offensive lump. Better in the warm climate, futile coughing followed by vomiting.

Hepar sulphuris: loose cough with bloody or thick yellow tenacious sputum, breathing difficulty on lying on the left side and aggravated on walking. Choking cough, rattling croaking cough, has to raise the head up, and bend the head backwards. Hep sulph follows Ant tart in Bronchopneumonia.

7 DERMATOLOGY

- Characteristic expressions of Skin in Psoric person
- Characteristic expressions of Skin in Sycotic person
- Characteristic expressions of Skin in Pseudopsoric person (Tubercular person)
- Characteristic expressions of Skin of Syphilitic person

Skin represents externally the inner turmoil that is happening in the body. These expressions on the skin differ from each other depending on the type of miasmatic qualities that an individual possesses. Hahnemann correlated this internal turmoil such as the haemorrhage, persistent local pains, abnormal local growths, the vertigo, the nervous attacks, the spasms, convulsions and many other expressions when he found that they disappear on the appearance of eruption on the skin. Based on the miasmatic considerations he classified them into three main categories: ***Psoric, Sycotic, Syphilitic.***

Pseudo-psoric or Tubercular classification is a post-Hahnemanian concept.

Characteristic expressions of Psora in skin condition:

Texture: dry, rough, dirty, or having an unhealthy look and unwashed appearance.

Anhidrosis: dry and unperspiring skin.

Pruritus: voluptuous itching and tickling. Rubs and scratches that relieves for few moment followed by long continued burning of the affected parts. Mostly late in the evening and at midnight. Pruritus can also occur in the disorders of the other systems without the involvement of the skin.

Discharge: scanty. Little suppuration, seropurulent, and occasionally bloody.

Eruptions: are often macular and papular with intense itching. Has only the colour of the skin unless there is secondary inflammatory process. The scales and the crusts are thin and fine almost on the affected parts.

Erysipelas: most commonly on the skin as a widespread erythema and cellulitis. Organisms gain entry into the skin through fissures in the skin, skin becomes red, swollen and tender. Constitutional symptoms like fever, malaise may accompany mostly due to streptococcal infection.

Pruritus: is a symptom and not a disease by itself. It is present in many conditions including Scabies, Atopic eczema, Candidiasis, Urticaria, insect bites etc. It may be present in systemic conditions even without obvious skin involvement. Metabolic disease, Malignant diseases, Haematological diseases, Renal and Liver diseases. Often Senile and Psychogenic conditions also present with lot of itching. Drugs reactions can also give these symptoms. It is obvious, therefore, for the treatment of the pruritus that the underlying cause need to be investigated. This pruritus can be of generalized nature or may be of local nature.

1. ***The patient reports with either generalized or local itching — may be of a recent origin or may be there for a few days. Itching provokes scratching at times, till it bleeds, the skin is hot and at times there is red discoloration. This may be present with or without eruption and with varying modalities. It is a case of PRURITUS.***

A detailed history, its onset and the course of itching, severity must be noted. Investigate any hyper-glycaemic state or any intake of drug for any other condition. Also note whether the patient is allergic to any physical, chemical or environmental factors.

Sulphur: is the first remedy that one can think of if the skin texture is dry, scaly and unhealthy, and little injury suppurates; freckles and voluptuous itching. Burning when scratched, and sensitive to air, wind, and washings. Eruptions are pimply, pustules and cracks, and excoriation in the fold. Itching aggravated by warmth. Even the varicose veins — when ulcerate and rupture — bleed.

Sulphur is potent antiseptic and one of the most important destroyer of scabies. But Sulphur has the property to repress the constitutional eruptions when locally applied, as well as the power to destroy the acarus. So Sulphur is given internally and oil of lavender is externally applied.

Sulphur has an independent antipsoric action beyond its property of bringing out the eruption. Psoric poison may be present active in a case and apparently well-indicated remedies fail to act in consequence.

Arsenic alb: has alternation with the internal problems or Asthma. The skin is dry scaly and shrivelled, worse in cold. When eruption is present they are papular, dry rough, scaly and worse by cold and scratching. Hives are aggravated by eating shell fish.

Itching, burning, swellings, oedema, spots, blue black white and pimples, vesicles burning violently. Free desquamation. Urticaria with burning and restlessness. Pustules turn malignant, wounds get easily poisoned and infected. Gangrene and carbuncles can develop easily.

Arsenic is closely connected to the cancerous diathesis, and it acts directly on the cancerous tissue and cancerous element and many cures have been reported by it in crude and in potencies. When subjective symptoms are present higher potencies work and the similarity is more crude or coarse, then the lower potencies are useful. Varicose veins burn like fire.

Rhus tox: has intense itching, the skin is dry, hot and burning. Tendency to form scales. Itch is aggravated by getting wet. Dermatitis, with intense itching, cellulitis with burning and eczematous eruption, with tendency to scale formation, sensitive to cold air.

Tendency to form vesicles and mostly the suppurative forms. And, therefore, indicated in shingles, herpes zoster, pempihigus. Urticarial rash is often present. Where the herpes alternates with asthma and dysentery, it is extremely useful.

Rhus venenata: has itching better by hot application. The skin is dark red, itching is more at night with pain in the long bones. There is tendency to erysipelas with dark red skin relieved by hot water.

Natrum mur: has herpetic eruptions. Itching is in the flexures, the skin is raw red and inflamed. Hives are itching and burning, worse by eating salt. Greasy skin. But dry eruptions on the margins of the hairy scalp and bends of the joint, behind the ears. Hives develop after exertion, with lot of burning and itching. Tendency to develop warts on the palms. It also affects the hair follicles causing alopecia. Redness of the old scar which are painful.

Dolichos pruriens: Has violent itching on the skin without any visible eruption or rash. Intense itching with no swelling or rash, more across the shoulder and hands, elbows and knees and the hairy part. The skin burns in the night when in bed.

2. ***Patient complains of intermittent transient swelling of the skin, brawny lesions around the lips and the orbit or genitalia and often associated with pruritus leaving to be normal in a short period of time. It is a case of URTICARIA.***

The most obvious homoeopathic remedy is **Urtica urens**. Burns and scalds with intense burning and itching. Hives with rheumatism after shellfish. Itching raises red blotches. Rheumatism alternates with nettle rash. In urticaria there is burning heat, with formication and violent itch. There is at times angio-neurotic oedema, herpes labialis with sensation of heat and itching.

Apis mel.: Develops sudden puffiness of the body with stinging pains. Skin is hot and dry with gushes of sweat. Carbuncle with burning. Apis has a slow action and it is beneficial if it is not changed soon. Increased flow of urine is a favorable picture.

Arsenic alb(see above): has urticaria with burning and restlessness, hives are worse on eating shelled fish. Some prescribers alternate Apis and Arsenic alb with beneficial results.

Chloralum hydratum: have red blotches like measles aggravated by spirituous liquors, hot drinks, often associated with palpitation. There is intense itching, surface of the body is stone cold. Chill brings on the wheals. Skin is sensitive, dry, yellow shriveled.

Antimonium crudum: is sensitive to cold bathing, develops measles-like eruption, white with red areola. Itching fearfully, particularly when getting warm in bed.

Aggravated at night. Eczema with gastric derangement, pimples, vesicles and pustules are very sensitive to cold bathing. Thick, hard, and honey-coloured scabs. Dry skin warts. Dry gangrene, scaly pustular eruption, with burning and itching. Develops callosities with slight pressure. Sensitive to cold, therefore suited to hydrogenoid constitution.

Antipyrinum: has swelling of lips, burning of mouth and gums, swollen tongue and, at times, there are some lumps in the cheek. On the skin intense itching, urticaria. Appearing and disappearing. There is erythema eczema, pemphigus. Angioneurotic oedema.

3. ***Patient presents with a very dry hot skin, with malaise and fever, rhinorrhoea, cough and conjunctival suffussion gradually increasing in intensity for the past two or three days. In all the probabilities the patient will break into rash on the skin. The condition is MEASLES.***

In **Aconite nap.:** there is dry burning heat in the nose, eyelids, mouth, throat, lungs and palms and wants to uncover. There is high fever with dry heat, red face, with mental anguish. Miliary eruption , maculo-papular rash, itching intense, often relieved by stimulants.

Bryonia: there is typical dryness of all the mucus membranes with hot dry skin, slow development of eruption of measles, the skin is yellow and pale, at times dropsical. Bryonia with other of its typical symptoms will help bring out the eruption of measles to full-blown picture. Bryonia may be continued till the eruption starts receding.

With more of conjunctival and nasal symptoms, **Cineraria** and **Euphrasia** eye drops are useful. If there is lot of itching in the eyes then **Arsenic alb** is very useful. Diarrhoea is a common complication of Measles and for that **Pulsatilla** is a good remedy. Similarly there is often a chest complication with a lot of congestion and cough and rattling in the chest.

Ant tart: very often this Ant Tart helps to bring out the suppressed eruption while resolving the chest condition. There is often troublesome cough without the chest involvement when **Kali bi.** is found very useful. (**See also chapter on Pyrexia**)

4. ***Patient, usually below 10 years of age, comes with sudden rise of temperature, reaching its pinnacle on the third day. The pulse is very fast, headache and muscular pain severe, vomiting initially, severe sore throat, with enlarged lymph glands, inflamed tonsils and pharynx with follicular exudate, red fauces, or scarlet in colour, flushed face, punctate rash that quickly spreads to the chest and hands within twenty-four hours, the tongue is strawberry coloured, characteristic desquamation that begins on the fourth day. The condition is SCARLATINA or SCARLET FEVER caused by haemolytic streptococcal eruption.***

With the introduction of Penicillin and improvement in the hygienic standards the episodes of scarletina have reduced considerably. Aconite and Belladonna look very close to the pathogenecity of Scarletina but they do not respond so well as they are expected to be.

Apis mel.: is the most remarkable remedy that helps here. There is scalding in the mouth and throat, swollen gums, swollen lips, tongue glossy as if varnished, red, shining and puffy. There are vesicles on the edge; better from cool air. Ulceration and the enlargement of glands which is a common accompaniment of scarletina. It is controlled by mercurius.

Mercurius: in many cases initially Rhus tox will be indicated and Lachesis may show up in later cases. Very severe form of scarletina with prominent general nervous toxication. Mercurius skin is moist, excessive odourous, viscid perspiration, and worse at night. Although there is perspiration patient does not feel relieved. Skin is yellow and excoriated like raw meat, there are pimples around the main eruption. Itching is worse from warmth. Ulcers are irregular and spreading, shallow, bleeding with proud flesh. Boils and abscess are formed at the time of menses. Great tendency to form pus.

Camphora: in repeated doses as a remedy similar to collapse state. Is suggested by Hartmann. If the collapse condition involves the brain then we should think of **Cuprum aceticum,** and **Zinc met.**

Ailanthus glandulosa: has better action than Arsenic and Lachesis. The symptoms are livid throat, rapid swelling, patchy eruption, with quick and feeble pulse, and oppressed brain. Low dilution of Ailanthus is preferred.

5. ***A patient comes with hot red skin, with oedema in the initial state, and intra-dermal vesicles: weeping or oozing of fluid on the surface, with formation of crusting in early stages and scaling in later stages, intense itching that produces excoriation, and later lichenification. This condition is DERMATITIS and ECZEMA.***

The meaning of word eczema is flowing over, which describes some of the above inlammatory changes — dermatitis. Both these words are used some what interchangeably.

Rhus tox: is the first remedy that one can think of. It has dry, red itching skin, worse on the hairy part. Burning eczematous eruption with tendency to scale formation. These are sensitive to cold air. Eruptions often alternate with dysentery. Many conditions are covered by this remedy, such as Shingles, Urticaria, Cellulitis, Pemphigus, Erysipelas, and other vesicular suppurative forms.

Antimonium crud: has sensitive pimples, vesicles and pustules to cold bathing. Urticaria and measles-like eruptions, white with red areola, with fearfull itching, develop when warm in bed. The skin is dry, with or without dry gangrene.

When skin is dry, scaly, unhealthy, and, when very little injury, suppurates with voluptuous itching, worse at night, heat of bed, scratching and washing. Burning when scratched — should remind one of Sulphur. Excoriation in the folds is characteristic. Frequent crops of boils, varicose veins are the characteristic. Scabies, eczema, ulcers, creeping erysipelas, excoriation on the folds fall under this category.

Arsenic alb: eruptions are dry rough scaly, parchment-like, worse from cold, and scratching. Free desquamation, Hives worse on eating shelled fish. Itching followed by burning, cutting pain followed by bloody offensive discharge. Many conditions like ulcers, pimpled vesicles, malignant pustules — Anthrax and poisoned wounds cover this.

6. ***An adolescent patient, roughly at puberty, presents with characteristic lesions of comedo a blackened horny follicular plug on the face, back, shoulders, the chest and on the back. The general skin is greasy, coarse and thickened with prominent follicular orifice. The condition is ACNE VULGARIS.***

Acne is formed because of the androgenic or eostrogenic influence in the young adult at puberty. An individual usually outgrows this condition but in some the condition may last for quite some times.

In a recent case of acne the eruption is red, with a small black head, often quite painful. If the patient is robust and full-blooded, he often needs **Belladonna.** The skin is quite glossy, dry and hot. There is often alternate redness and paleness of the skin. Associated with this, generalized boils develop.

But if the patient is pale and slender the picture of **Pulsatilla** is evident. The other constitutional characteristics of Pulsatilla should be present. The development of acne is mostly during puberty and nearing the menses.

In chronic cases, when the indicated remedy does not act or when there is recurrence of these eruptions, then one should think of **Sulphur**. After every crop of acne they tend to disappear without leaving any tell-tale marks.

But few of them may suppurate with a lot of pain, very sensitive to touch and bleed easily. The skin is unhealthy and easily suppurates. This is **Hepar sulphuris**.

When there is induration of the acne — bluish red skin, worse on the face and chest, often pustular, intense itching leaving a scar on the skin after the eruption. **Kali bromatum** is indicated. The general tendency of the skin is to cause boils and indolent painful pustules. Generalised pimples and pustules on the skin and face, mostly painless, but they bleed when scratched — **Calcarea sulph.**

Characteristic expression of sycosis in the skin condition.

Greasy oily skin.

Pruritus , in the folds of the limbs and the genitals, and along the line of the hair. Eruptions patchy, circumscribed.

Cicatrices : Scarring, wounds burn and scald, insect bites. Abscesses.

7. ***The child has developed erythema, a weeping eruption or scaling on the face and has been gradually spreading over the other sites of the body. It is either an ENDOGENOUS ECZEMA OR ATOPIC DERMATITIS.***

This starts in the first three months of life in about 75% of children, mostly on the cheek, sparing the nose and central face. Seborrhoeic dermatitis of the scalp precedes the infantile eczema of the face. Erythema, exudation, and crusting, later spreads to the extensor surface of the limbs. This aggravates in the colder months, during teething and gastrointestinal disturbances. It is observed that it exists more in the unfavourable and unhealthy home atmosphere. With increasing age, say 13-15 years, the chances of getting skin lichenified increases and weeping nature of the skin stops. It may gradually transform into bronchial asthma. It is an inborn constitutional state, and is inherited. They are more susceptible to various food and eggs. It may start with physical trauma during washing with soap, cloth, woollens, and rapid changes of temperature.

Rhustox: skin is dry, red and intense itching, hot and burning, and the eruption is more on the hairy part. There is cellulitis, burning eczematous, eruption with tendency to scale formation. Sensitive to cold air eruptions alternate, with dysentery. Pus erodes the hair. Vesicles are formed over the abscesses. The onset is redness and swelling of the affected part with intolerable itching and burning, agglutination of the lids follow after sleep. After a while the skin gets studded with confluent bullae where the cellular tissue is loose. This dermatitis soon starts looking like erysipelas, and the whole face gets involved.

Rhus venanata: the skin is dark and red erysipelas. The vesicles are formed with nightly itching and pains in the long bones. It is also found very useful in pemphigus. Usually the lower potency is found useful.

Arsenic alb: the skin is dry, rough and shrivelled, worse by cold and scratching. Eruptions are papular, lot of itching and burning. Free desquamation. The skin symptoms are aggravated by eating shell-fish.

Psorinum: herpetic eruptions on the scalp and bends of the limbs, with lot of itching. The skin is oily and formation of indolent ulcers. The eruption is marked behind the ears. The skin is rough, scabby and greasy, intolerable itching, aggravated by the heat of the bed.

Vinca minor: eczema is mostly on the head and face, with corrosive itching. Great sensitiveness of the skin. The pustules are burning, itching, with offensive odour. Weeping eczema intermingled with foul thick crust.

8. ***Patient has almost persistent erythema, accompanied by profuse and repeated exfoliation. This includes nails and hair. There are enlarged lymph nodes, complains of constant cold. This is EXFOLIATIVE DERMATITIS.***

The entire skin is erythematous, oedematous and scaly. Mostly it is idiopathic without a preceding skin condition or it may follow dermatitis, psoriasis, or other skin conditions. It can also be a reaction to many drugs e.g. sulphonamides, sulphonylureas, gold. It can occasionally be the feature of systemic disorders like lymphomas.

Kali arsenicosum: the patient has a tendency to anxiety and skin diseases. Restless, nervous and anaemic. More useful when the patient's condition is moving towards malignancy. All the sufferings are worse at night. There is intolerable itching, worse from undressing and application of warmth and walking. Fissures on the bend of the arm, knees. Skin has tendency to cancer, and sets in without any signs and symptoms.

Berberis aquafolia: eruption on the scalp, extending to face and neck. At times the eruption is dry, pruritus is located in localized spots initially and then spreads over the whole skin. Appear as rashes, blisters, pustules, papules, and urticarious itching, better by washing in the cold water.

Hydrocotyle asiatica: it shows excessive thickening of the skin, copper-coloured eruption in various places. Intolerable itching, especially of the soles and vagina. Skin has dry eruption, great thickening of the epidermal layer and shows exfoliation of the scales, is, therefore, useful in Psoriasis, Acne, Elephantiasis. Yellowish spots on the legs and pricking in the different parts with itching in the various places. Useful in great variety of skin disorders like acne, eczema, pemphigus, lupus, copper-coloured eruption, with intolerable itching in various places.

Petroleum: eczema with deep cracks in the folds, nipples, finger-tips, itching at night, itching orifices with burning, chilblains with moist itch and burn, the skin is hard, dry, rough, thickened like parchment. Skin gets raw, festers or will not heal. Smallest of the scratch suppurates. Thick greenish crust, burning and itching. Red, raw and cracks easily, cracks worse in winter. The skin is extremely sensitive to touch of the clothes.

Graphites: eczema is dry, rough, irritable but breaks easily and oozes out exudate, gluey moisture, worse in the folds and heals slowly. Moist crusty eruption. Phlegmonous erysipelas of the face, burning and stinging pains.

9. ***Patient presents with the lesion on the scalp showing diffused scaling and erythema, spreading over the eyebrows, naso-labial folds, ears and neck. There are some papules and pustules. The skin looks greasy and scaly. The condition is SEBORRHOEIC DERMATITIS.***

It affects those areas of the skin where there is a high density of sebaceous glands. The cause is unknown. Neurogenic factor may play a part.

The scalp is primarily involved that shows diffused scaling and erythema. Other sites may be involved like sternal region, thoracic spine, para-spinal skin, the axillae, the groin folds, and perianal region. With more severe and acute state, the skin looks more greasy, scales, weeping and maceration.

Application of Lotion of Calendula mother tincture with Staphysagria mother tincture in equal proportion is found beneficial.

Mezereum: the patient is very sensitive to cold air. Ill-effects suppressed eczema, capitis vaccination and mercurial poisoning. The eruptions ooze acrid gluey moisture from thick crusts, scabs with pus beneath. Deep hard painful ulcers, worse by touch and warmth. Intolerable itching which is worse by warmth and in bed. Itching changes the place of scratching. Ulcers itch and burn surrounded by pustules and vesicles. Senile pruritus.

Thuja: never well since vaccination, skin troubles and neuralgia follow. Eruptions itch or burn violently, worse on cold bathing. Eruptions are mostly on the covered parts, worse after scratching. Skin is very sensitive to touch. Nails get crippled, brittle and soft. Luxuriant growth of hair on the skin normally devoid of hair.

Vinca Minor: there is eczema of the head and face. Corrosive itching. Sensitiveness of the skin, red and sore from slight rubbing. Pustules itch, burn and emanate offensive odour. Hair gets matted together. Weeping eczema intermingled with foul thick crust.

Mercurius: constantly moist skin, excessive odourous, viscid perspiration, Although there is perspiration in excess there is no relief to the patient. Pimples around the main eruption itching worse from warmth. Yellowish-brown crust, considerable suppuration. Ulcers are irregular, spreading, shallow, bleeding, with cutting and proud flesh. Boils and abscess are more nearing the menses.

10. ***Patient presents with well-demarcated salmon pink lesions surrounded by silvery scaling, mostly over the extensor surfaces of the limb, elbows and knee. There may be many minor scattered hyperkeratic scales. The condition is PSORIASIS.***

Psoriasis is one of the most commonest disorders of the skin which occurs between the age of 10 and 30. The cause is not known. But it is a multi-miasmatic expression.

Genetic factors are very important in the aetiology of this disease. The role of infection is the exacerbation factor. Lesion are mostly on the trunk and limbs. Emotional trauma is the most important factor since many skin disease are of nervous origin. Mechanical trauma to the skin on the elbows and the lumbar area in sedentary people. Psoriasis presents with different form-flexural psoriasis, pustular and nail involvement.

Arsenic Iod: marked exfoliation of the skin, in large scales, leaving raw exuding surface beneath. Enlarged scrofulous glands,watery oozing from the eczema of the beard, itching worse on washing. The discharges from the mucus membrane are persistently acrid, profuse, thick, gluey. Better in open air.

Chrysarobinum: the lesions are vesicular or squamous, associated with foul smelling discharge and crust formation. These tend to become confluent and give the appearance of one big area — there is violent itching of thighs, legs and around ears. Eczematous eruption behind the ears, very useful in psoriasis and ringworm.

Graphites: dry, rough, irritable skin developing eczema, that breaks easily and exudes a gluey moisture. Slow to heal. Burning in old scars and they ulcerate. There are also moist and crusty eruptions, when the skin is very unhealthy.

Hydrocotyle: great thickening of epidermoid layer, and exfoliation of the skin. Intolerable itching, specially of the soles. Pustules on the chest.

Kali arsenicum: there is intolerable itching, usually after undressing. Chronic eczema itching is worse from warmth, walking, undressing.

11. ***A middle-aged person gives a history of pain, tingling, and dysaesthesia, along the course of the nerve with appearance of characteristic eruption(vesicles, papules, bullous lesion) throughout the dermatome. This condition is SHINGLES or HERPES ZOSTER.***

Varicella zoster virus is responsible for this condition. The dorsal root ganglia of certain cranial nerves pick up the original infection of an attack of chicken pox many years previously. The viruses of chicken pox and herpes zoster are identical.

Much before the virus reemerges in the skin, many days preceding the appearance of vesicles, papules, bullous lesions on the entire dermatome appear. The whole presents three sets of symptoms: The pain that starts much before the appearance of vesicles; actual eruption vesicles, and later pustules follow — with severe itching .

Homoeopathic remedies will depend upon the stage of the disease and symptoms presented.

Ranunculus bulbosus: the pains are stitching, stabbing, shooting, extort tears, with shuddering. Restless, cannot stay in one position. Often accompanied by burning, bruised soreness. Sensitive to air and touch. In due course it develops small, deep, transparent, dark blue little elevated blisters the size of an ordinary pinhead.

Rhus tox: there is dry, hot, burning itching, and is worse on hairy parts. Develops cellulitis burning eczematous eruption, and vesicular suppurative form. Very sensitive to cold air. Pus erodes the hair. Vesicles are formed over the abscesses. There are neuralgic pains along the dermatome that corresponds to the pathogenesis of Herpes.

Tarentula cubens: it affects the cellular tissue, and, therefore, useful in septic condition. Although the incubation is slow, the condition progresses rapidly with alarming proportion: atrocious burning. There is itching around genitals, purplish hue and burning stinging pains. Also useful in carbuncles — bluish abscesses which are painful.

Arsenic alb.: skin is dry, rough and scaly and looks like parchment. There is itching, burning and swelling. Pimples burn and itch, free desquamation. Burning pains are the characteristics of Arsenic, that are better by warm application.

Post-herpes pains in the elderly are common. Although the original infection settles down, secondary infection can cause lot of discomfort. The neuralgic pains start in the same nerve where the shingles had developed.

Mezereum and Rhus tox are two remedies which are found useful in post-herpetic neuralgia.

12. ***Patient reports with widespread, highly irritant, excoriated, secondarily infected, folliculo-papular eruption in the finger webs, wrist, elbows, ankles, breast, and genitals. The condition is mostly SCABIES.***

Transmission of this infection is by skin to skin contact, with an affected individual, and this occurs in bed. Warmth is necessary for the acarus or the mite to remain mobile and thereby pass from one to other. The important sites where these mites burrow are finger web, elbows, ankles, breast, and genitals. They develop widespread, highly irritating excoriation, and often secondary infected folliculo-papular eruption. The itching is severe when papules appear over genitals, and children develop these papules on the palms, soles, and in axillary folds.

Sulphur: is the primary remedy but it may not be the only remedy to start with. Unless the totality of sulphur is present it may not work. No doubt it is a great anti-psoric remedy. Eruptions are almost of every kind and they alternate with other complaints, asthma etc. It is an unhealthy skin which breaks out and festers and takes long to heal. Very dry, unhealthy, scaly skin, every little injury suppurates, voluptuous itching, worse at night, and heat of bed. Scratching induces burning.

Psorinum: Hering prepared this nosode from the sero-purulent matter of scabies vesicles. Useful in chilly patients and when there is lack of reaction in chronic diseases, well-related remedies fail to relieve or cure, and most important — when sulphur feels indicated but fails to react. Psorinum chiefly affects the skin folds, axillae, first in the left then in the right. It has also marked action on the allergic state. The skin is dirty, rough and scabby, greasy, breaks out in folds, intolerable itching, worse on heat of the bed, scratches till it bleeds. Eruptions look like herpetic eruption in the folds and bends of joints, with itching. Sebaceous glands secrete excessively, indulent ulcers, slow to heal, eruptions are crusty, skin is oily. Excrescences disappear in summer and they reappear in winter. Recurring body lice, scabies, condylomata, developing on the edges of the skin.

Sepia: the skin texture is rough, hard, or cracked. They are worse in the flexures. Herpetic eruption on the lips, about mouth and nose. Thick crusts are on the elbows, ulcers on small joints. Ringworm in isolated parts, and they appear always in spring. Scratching does not relive itching. Urticarial rash is worse in open air, and is better in warm room. Hyperdrosis, and bromidrosis, sweat on feet, worse on toes, and a very intolerable odour.

Hepar sulphuris: Hepar has very unhealthy skin, very little injury suppurates, very sensitive to slightest touch, chapped skin with deep cracks on hand and feet. Papules are prone to suppurate, and extend. Very sensitive to cold, cannot bear to be uncovered, and wants to be wrapped. Ulcers are very sensitive to contact, burning, stinging, and easily bleed. Putrid ulcers are surrounded by little pimples.

Very sensitive to cold, chill and liability to catch cold.

Mercurius: constantly moist skin, with viscid perspiration, but there is no relief from this perspiration. Eruptions are vesicular and pustular, skin is tender like raw meat, pimples around the main eruption. Itching is worse from warmth of the bed. Eczema is moist, crusta lactea, with yellowish-brown crust, with considerable suppuration. Ulcers are irregular, spreading. Bleeding like cutting the proud flesh. Boils and abscesses form during the menses. It has a tendency to form pus — mostly in the cavities of abscesses, which burn and sting.

Graphites : like Sulphur it is a great anti-psoric too. The skin of graphites is rough, dry and hard. Eczematous and herpetic eruptions predominate. Eruptions on the occiput exuding gluey humor. Eczema of the ear, moist eczema round the anus, pimples etc. There is ulceration of the old scars, which burn.

13. ***A young individual presents with papular lesions that are coarse and roughened surfaces developing on a palmar aspect of the fingers, neck, and knees. The condition is WARTS.***

This is a viral infection caused by human papilloma virus. These also infect the domestic animals. These viruses affect the various sites and these warts are known by the sites on which they erupt. e.g. when they are seen on the soles are known as plantar warts, when they are on the face, neck, nose etc. they are known as filiform warts, and genital warts are super-infected with venereal transmission.

The repertories will give different rubrics such as excrescences, condylomata, and warts If we see the remedies under these rubrics they are not very different.

Under warts there are sub-rubrics describing the color, site, shape, consistency etc. Remedies frequently indicated are **Thuja, Causticum, Nitric acid, Dulcamara,** and **Antim crud.** But while taking the history of the patient, it will be necessary to inquire into all other aspects which are mentioned under sub-rubrics. In addition to these local symptoms of the wart, it is necessary to take the general symptoms of the patient.

Thuja: it acts mainly on the mucous membranes of genito-urinary tract, intestines, skin . Thuja has the formation of wart-like growths upon mucous membrane and skin surfaces. Fig warts and condylomata. It is for soft, exuberant fungoid tissue polyps condylomata and warts pedunculated, black, suppressed. The eruptions itch or burn violently, worse on cold bathing.

Causticum: the skin is of a dirty white shallow complexion, with warts especially on the face. Warts are seedy, large and jagged, bleeding easily, ulcerating on the finger, nose, eye-lids.

Nitric acid: the action of Nitric acid is mostly on the muco-cutaneous junction. The warts are large, jagged, bleed on touch or washing. Sensitive and splinter-like pains, zigzag irregular edges, base looks like raw flesh.

Dulcamara: the warts are large smooth, on face, and palmar surface of the hands. Pruritus if any gets aggravated in cold and wet weather. It is a scrofulous remedy and has many scrofulous-looking eruptions, moist or dry, red tettery eruptions, specially on face, warts are fleshy and large and smooth.

Antimonium crud.: scaly pustular eruptions with burning and itching, callosities from slight pressure. There is dry skin.

14. ***Child presents with discoid patch and slight swelling, and vasculisation of adjoining borders usually on a non-hairy part of the body. Itching at times. This is TINEA CIRCINATA or common ringworm.***

Tinea is formed in the different parts of the body and they are then termed according to their site. T. pedis, T. curare T. capitis etc. Tinea means 'moth-eaten'. The source of this fungus is zoophilic — Animal to man; anthrophilic — man to man; and geophilic — soil to man.

The disease varies with the site of the infection. When the infection is in the foot, it may present with fissuring of the toe webs, scaling of the plantar surface, or vesicles around the toe web. The inter-digital lesions may be pruritic, and with the superinfection of bacteria there could be pain. In the scalp there can be alopecia, and scaling.

Sepia: ringworm-like eruptions develop every spring, itching is not relieved by scratching. Worse in bends of elbows and knees. The vesicles itch, thick crusts form on the joints. Sweat on the feet, worse on toes, intolerable odour. Ringworm on the face, every spring, roundness and yellowness of the parts. The itching is desperate, particular when it is on the genitals and anus.

Tellurium: itching of hands and feet, face, worse on whole body lower limbs, infection on the chin known as Barber's itch, offensive odour, patches are circular, mostly on the scalp, back of ears, small red patches, circular in shape, itching is worse in cool air.

Sulphur: the skin infection is almost every type, and these eruptions alternate with other complaints. Eruptions are pimply, pustules, crack hand-nails. It is always preferred to give Sulphur internally than as an ointment as an external application because it is seen that it represses the infection.

For these skin infections one should try and prescribe the constitutional remedy because the skin infection is often the result of suppressed internal turmoil.

Arsenicum iodatum: is the first rank remedy that one should think of. The skin is dry, scaly and itching. There is marked exfoliation of the skin, large scales, leaving a raw exuding surface beneath. Often there is voluptuous itching and the scratch marks leave behind hard horny surface. These get aggravated by mental exertion.

Characterisic expressions of Tubercular Miasm: Pseudo-psoric:

Tubercular eruptions look like unwashed, dirty, skin with pronounced pruritus.

Eruptions are vesicular, pustular. Skin texture is greasy oily.

Excessive, offensive perspiration.

Glandular involvement.

15. ***Patient complains of aching pains and sense of tiredness in the legs, at times irritation and discoloration of the site over the distended vein, oedema around the ankle, at the end of the day. Varicose veins may develop with eczema and ulceration. The condition is THROMBOPHLEBITIS / (VARICOSE ULCERS).***

Varicose veins are caused because of incompetent valves at long saphino-femoral or popliteal junction or when the valves of the communicating veins joining the superficial and deep veins are deficient so that the blood drains from deep veins into superficial vessels.

Hamamelis virginiana: the principal action of this remedy is on the veins, of the genitals, limbs, and throat, producing venous congestion, varicose veins, haemorrhoids, and haemorrhages. On the skin there is ecchymosis, traumatic inflammation, bluish chilblains, phlebitis, varicose veins and ulcers. There is great lassitude and weariness of the limbs and elsewhere very sore muscles. Neuralgia of the long saphenous nerve.

Fluoricum acid: has intense soreness. Its action is on the ulcers and varicose veins apart from the action on the bones. It is typically an anti-tubercular and anti-syphilitic drug which shows the haemorrhagic and destructive nature. The parts are better from cold water washing and better by walking in the open air.

Vipera berus/Vipera torva.: the keynote of Vipera in cases of phlebitis and varicose veins, is worse on letting the limb hang down as if it would burst with fullness. It has also action on the veins. Shuffling gait formed by the paralysis of the foot. Better by elevating the foot.

Apart from the medication, stretchable socks or spiral stretchable bandage should be tried and standing job should be prohibited.

16. ***Patient is a child, develops thin-walled vesicles, on the erythematous base, on the face, neck and scalp, often extending peripherally in the center. The exuding serum forms a yellow-brown crust. There is no fever but lymphadenitis may be present. There may be history of earlier pediculosis, scabies or other skin diseases. The condition is IMPETIGO CONTAGIOSA.***

Repertory describes different remedies under different head of sites. Baring few changes the remedies are the same.

Antimonium crud: pimples, pustules, and boils are on the face. The eruption is yellow-crusted, on the cheeks and chin. Small sores, honey-coloured granules on chin.

These are sensitive to cold bathing. Thick, hard and honey-coloured scabs. Eczema with gastric derangement.

Echinacea angustifolia: recurring boils, carbuncles, little papules on the skin with redness, feeling like nettle, mostly on the face and neck.

17. ***The patient has hypopigmented skin patches associated with loss of sensation to touch or temperature with nerve involvement (Thickening or tenderness). Complains of transient rash, with features of acute febrile illness. It is a case of LEPROSY.***

Leprosy is another destructive process of tubercular origin and it can cause vicious and unprecedented deformity. It happens mostly in persons of lymphatic temperament where these destructive processes start in advanced age. It is in the tubercular miasm that we have to face so much difficulty in eradicating these conditions.

Huges mentions two remedies which Nureing used and treated some cases successfully — *Gynocardia odorate*, common name **'Chaulmoogra'** and *Dipterocarpus turbinatus*, common name **'Gurjun'.** The oils are derived from these plants. In fact, apart from this information we do not have much to work on. Nureing is reported to have treated many cases and claims to cure some of those.

Hydrocotyle asiatica: Indian pennywort, produces hypertrophy and induration of connective tissue. Boileau used it first as remedy for leprosy. The pathogenesis suggest the similarity of lepra, it is considered to be one of the remedies for leprosy.

18. ***A patient between the age of 50-60 develops insidiously persistent bright red sore, denuded mucosa, flaccid bullae, forming soft crust on the scalp much before the generalized bullous eruption. The bullae erupt leaving raw moist area. These walled blisters are elsewhere on the body too. This condition is PEMPHIGUS.***

Pemphigus is a rare disease, in which an antibody, usually of the IgG class, reacts with the antigen at the surface of the epidermal cells that form part of the intercellular cement substance.

There are several forms of pemphigus. In the most common form, lesions may be confined to the mucosal surface in the early stages of the disease. The sites can vary — it may be on the skin and in the mouth. Lesions rupture to leave moist eroded areas. Secondary bacterial infection is common.

Caltha palustris: marsh marigold is a plant belonging to Ranunculaceae, and the tincture is made from the fresh shoots and flowers. However, it is an unproved drug. Hensen gives its indications "Pemphigus bullae are surrounded by a ring, much itching, on the third day they are transformed into crusts ".

Ranunculus scleratus: most acrid plant in the Ranunculi family. Causing burning in the mouth, throat, stomach, chest, urethra, other parts. It is well-proved drug. The skin has yellow vesicular eruptions, with tendency to form large blisters, acrid exudation which make the surrounding part sore. Most of the symptoms are right-sided except one gnawing sensation in the left arm. It has mapped and peeled tongue associated with smarting and burning and boring pains.

Manicinella: has intense erythema. Vesicles, large blisters as from scald. Fungoid growth, with heavy brown crusts with extensive blisters oozing of sticky serum and formation of crusts. Low potencies are useful.

19. *Middle-aged woman, apparently with lot of tension and of nervous temperament, shows on the skin characteristic lesions of shining flat topped polygonal papules, dull ink or violet in colour, moderate to severely irritable at the onset, usually on the flexure surfaces of the wrist, forearm, around the waist, inner surfaces of the thigh, and the lower legs which are often hypertrophic, large and horny. The condition is LICHEN PLANUS.*

Antimonium crudum: scaly, pustular eruptions, with burning and itching worse at night. Slight pressure causes callosities. Thick hard honey-coloured scabs Stomach symptoms are very important, are associated with the skin symptoms. Many effects are because of suppressed eruptions.

Arsenic alb.: with all the charcteristics of lichen planus there is burning .of skin. Arsenic is very potent and has deep action on the economy.

Jugulans cinarea: it has many types of skin symptoms. Skin looks red like scarlatina. Itching and pricking when heated. The pustules are mostly on the lower extremities.

20. ***Patient complains of localized or widespread eruption of wheals preceded and accompanied by severe itching. There may be no lesion when examined. It is probably URTICARIA.***

Urticaria is considered more a multimiasmatic trait but pseudopsora predominates.

In a case of acute urticaria, the cause can be frequently established but in a case of chronic urticaria the cause often remains unknown.

The common causes are food allergy — shellfish allergy is the commonest. Usually the gastrointestinal symptoms are associated.

Drug allergy: drugs like penicillin and serum sickness are the commonest.

Other factors are:

Parasites, intestinal worms, amoebiasis.

Bacterial infection.

Physical factors like light, cold, heat or exertion.

Psychogenic factors are most important.

Apis mellifica: the well-known effect of the bee sting, burning stinging sharp pains, excessive swelling because of serous fluid collection gives the leading key-notes for its employment in great many conditions. Oedematous swelling, sudden puffiness of the whole body, swelling developing after bites or sting. Rosy red, sensitive sore skin with stinging pains. Skin is dry hot, alternating with gushes of sweat. Great anxiety, restlessness, and fidgety with allergic oedema. Better from cool air, cold bathing, uncovering. Worse from touch and pressure.

Natrum mur: it is chronic of Apis and is useful in many cases of skin eruptions. The hives develop after exertion, with lot of itching and burning. The psychologic reasons of developing the eruptions on the skin are more common. It covers the effects of grief, disappointments, depressed and introverted and one who dwells on past unpleasant memories. Consolation aggravates.

Urtica urens: is a stinging nettle that produces stinging burning pains. Develops hives with rheumatism after shell-fish, with pinworms. Itching and raised blotches, the eruption can appear periodically every year. The skin has burning heat, with formication, violent itching. This can be consequence of the suppressed nettle rash and the rheumatism alternating with nettle rash. Often angio-neurotic odema develop. Gout and rheumatism are associated with urticaria-like eruption.

Bovista : On excitement develops urticaria with rheumatic lameness, palpitation and diarrhoea. The whole body is covered with itching urticaria. Skin complaints when not relieved by Rhus tox, Bovista helps.

Characteristic expressions of the syphilitic miasm

Pruritus negligible.

Tumors over growths, condylomata.

Gangrene.

21. ***A patient with one or more fingers, or the toes, perhaps part of the hand or foot, complains of cold, and looks purple and shrivelled and evokes a characteristic odour and loss of sensation but severe pain in the adjoining living tissue with or without secondary infection. It is GANGRENE.***

Mostly two types of Gangrene are known. The most common is invariably due to arterial block. The extremities become white, cold and anaesthetic. Soon it becomes painful and gradually becomes dry and mummified. As thrombosis slowly extends up the limb the gangrene spreads until a line of demarcation forms where an adequate blood supply is reached. The commonest type is senile gangrene due to arteriosclerosis.

Moist gangrene occurs when the part is engorged with blood and is aggravated when there is arterial occlusion, is combined with venous occlusion; the result of thrombosis, pressure, injury or inflammation. Usually we find this on the feet of diabetics.

Gas gangrene is due to infection and necrosis of muscles, by spore-forming anaerobic organisms.

Anthracinum: this nosode is very valuable remedy in malignant or septic inflammations of connective or cellular tissues. It forms carbuncles, abscesses and boil-like eruptions and malignant ulcers. Gangrene is with foul secretions, ulcerations are sloughing, and intolerable burning. Restless and debilitated.

Arsenic alb.: pains of the ulcer are burning, relieved by heat. Seaside complaints. Pains are maddening, burning like fire, hot needles or wires. Restless, and sudden great weakness.

Cantheris: its action is rapid and intense and the inflammations are violently acute or rapidly destructive — in the mucus and serous membranes. Produces most violent inflammation. Tendency to gangrene.

Lachesis: skin has bluish purplish appearance, blisters become dark, with black edges. There is purpura with intense prostration. Capillaries are dilated and small wounds bleed much.

Secale cornutum: it is a vegetable nosode. It has action on the vasomotor, where there is first contraction and then dilatation of blood vessel, the fingers turn blue and black. This stagnation leads to dry gangrene of the part. Secale shrivels up the skin, makes it dry and produces harsh shallow complexion. It lessens the coagulating property and produces the haemorrhagic diathesis, persistent offensive bleeding. It is worse by external heat but there is already an internal heat. There is tingling as if ants are crawling; better by rubbing.

Tarentula cubens: it is suited for severe septic conditions, alarming prostration, atrocious burning, sharp stinging pains and board-like hardness of affected parts.

22. ***A young woman complains of one or more fingers going suddenly dead, for an hour or more, occurs symmetrically on both the sides, especially in cold weather : in a long-standing case an ulcer may form on the tip of the finger. The condition is RAYNAUD'S DISEASE.***

Raynaud's phenomena consists of spasms of the arteries supplying the fingers or toes, is usually precipitated by cold and relieved by heat. When this Raynaud's Phenomena occurs without any underlying cause it is known as Raynaud's Disease. It is usually bilateral, and fingers are affected more commonly than the toes. Numbness and burning of the fingers usually occurs and the pain can be severe. Between the attacks the pulse and the digits appear normal. But in persistent and severe case there is possibility that gangrene can develop.

Agaricus muscarius: there is weakness in the loins, uncertain gait, trembling, itching of the toes, and feet as if frozen. Cramp in the soles of the feet Pain in the shin bone. Numbness of feet on crossing them. Tearing painful contractures in the calves.

Rhus tox, Sepia, Silicea have their own pathogenecity and does not need an explanation.

8 DISEASES OF BONES, JOINTS AND CONNECTIVE TISSUE

- Acute Osteomyelitis
- Osteoporosis
- Osteomalecia
- Olecranon Bursitis
- Frozen Shoulder
- Acute rheumatism
- Rheumatoid Arthritis
- Osteoarthritis
- Lumbago
- Cervical Spondylosis

1. ***A young person, after suffering a local injury, comes with severe pain and extreme local tenderness, starting near the end of a long bone, pus making its way to the surface under the periosteum with local swelling, redness and heat. There is a marked temperature around 104° F. The condition is ACUTE OSTEOMYELITIS.***

Acute osteomyelitis is often due to coagulase-positive staphylococcus arising from the focus on the skin, in the tonsils or from the wound. At times pneumococci or H. influenzae is responsible. The infection is due to bacteraemia. A small abscess is formed which makes its way up towards the surface under the periosteum or occasionally in the medulla of the bone.

Calcarea Phos: suited to delicate and tall thin children, scrofulous and of gouty constitution. Bones are osteoporus, slow ossification, non-union of bones, rickets. This is typically tubercular constitution, and is prescribed on the constitutional expression.

Fluoricum acidum: it has an action on the long bones causing decay and necrosis and favours the expulsion of the necrosed part. Destructiveness is the key-note of this acid and produces slow deep destructive effects. The patient is compelled to move about energetically. The tissues are puffy, indurated, and fistulous. Discharges are thin, foul, acrid, causing itching. Fluoric acid is hot patient and always better by cold.

Aurum metallicum: Aurum is suited to sanguine people with syphilitic and mercurial traits when implanted on to scrofulous characters. Destruction of bones is like secondary syphilis. Pains in bones are mostly at night. Bones of head, lumps under the scalp, exostosis, decay of nasal, palatine and mastoid bones fall under its influence. Soreness of the affected bones, better in open air, and are worse at night. Paralytic and tearing pains in the joints. There is cold foul sweat in the feet. Boring pains and burning stitches predominate.

Mezerium: it is a vegetable analogue and is most important antidote to mercurius. Mezerium affects the skin, bones, nerves, and mucous membranes and is very sensitive to cold air. Decay and exostosis of bones, periostitis, and bones seem enlarged. The secretions are acrid and has lot of pus. Bones, specially the long bones are inflamed, and swollen, develop decay and exostosis; the pains are worse at night. Burning in tibia and in the long bones. From the eruption that develops over the osteomyelitic area, ooze acrid gluey moisture, often green in colour, form a thick crust, scabs with pus beneath. The ulcer is thick and hard and painful.

Silicea: useful in diseases of bones and cartilages, decay and necrosis. Softening of bones. Silica can stimulate the organism to reabsorb fibrotic conditions and scar tissues. It is related to all pustulous burrowings — Felons, abscesses, boils, old scar ulcers. It promotes expulsion of foreign bodies. In osteomyelitis, the pus and the sequestrum formed by the decay and necrosis of the bone.

Gunpowder: it is mixture of Carbon-sulphur-kali nitricum. Gun-powder is for healing the wounds which refuse to heal. Also is a very good remedy for acute infections, boils, abscesses and bites. It has antiseptic properties. Low potency of Gun-powder is used.

2. ***Post-menopausal woman or an elderly man complains of low back pain which is occasionally more severe with a minor fall or an injury. The condition may be OSTEOPOROSIS.***

Osteoporosis is the reduced bone mass per unit bone volume. This leads to reduced strength and increased risk of fracture often with even a minor trauma. The bone mass decreases with increasing age and osteoporosis is commonest in post-menopausal women as oestrogen prevents bone resorption. This group is more prone to fractures specially Colles, neck of the femur, and vertebral sites.

Calcarea carb, and Calcarea phos: are two major remedies for this condition. This will promote the absorption of calcium from the food that the patient takes. But all the same it will be necessary to supplement large doses of calcium and vitamin D for early benefit. High consumption of milk is advised. Apart from this it is necessary to determine the constitutional remedy so that it can be given intermittently during the course of the treatment.

3. ***An adult presents with bone and muscle pain and tenderness, often due to sub-clinical fracture and the signs of proximal myopathy with a characteristic waddling gait. The condition is OSTEOMALACIA.***

Asafoetida: the pains in the limb, particularly in the tibia, are intolerable and are mostly at night. There is severe backache, preventing any work. Cold swelling around the ankle. Painful periosteum, swollen and enlarged. Decay of bones and deep ulceration producing thin ichorous pus. The pains are pressive, sharp, stitching and extending outwards, associated with numbness. Pains change place and are better by touch.

Mercurius vivus: patient is very sensitive to cold. Bone pains deep ,or near the surface. Worse at night. Must go out and walk about. Trembling limbs, especially the hands, as in Parkinson's disease. Lacerating pains in the joints. Dropsical swelling of the feet and legs. There is a sensation as if the knees are larger.

4. ***Patient complains of sudden pain in the elbow after an history of repeated trauma with slight swelling and tenderness. The condition is OLECRANON BURSITIS.***

There are numerous bursae around the body and any of these can become inflamed. They may appear for no obvious reasons or they may be secondary to trauma, repetitive injury, or arthritis. In many cases no treatment is required but only protection to the inflamed site.

Ruta: is one of the chief remedies for injuries of joints, tendons, bones and bursae. Pains are bruised. Complains from straining flexor tendons, bursitis with cracking in joints; worse walking in open air.

Bellis perennis: muscular and joint rheumatism, post-traumatic and rheumatic myalgic pains. Joints are sore. Muscular soreness. Wrist feels contracted as from elastic band. Better from continued motion, cold application. Worse from cold and immobility, sprains and injuries.

Lycopersicum: intense aching, rheumatic pain in the muscles of all limbs, with lame and tired feeling. Sharp pain on the right deltoid and pectoral muscles, worse lifting arm upwards and outwards.

Bryonia: swelling of elbow, every spot is painful on pressure. Along with typical bryonia symptoms.

5. ***Patient complains of unilateral pain the shoulder, at times in both the shoulders, with radiation of pain to the arm, aggravated at night. The condition is FROZEN SHOULDER.***

It is a common condition occurring in adults at any age. In most cases this condition appears without any obvious cause, but it can be occasionally related to overuse or injury. There is restriction in the glenohumeral movement. In a mild case simple exercises can correct the situation. Physiotherapy is the best solution apart from some minor medication.

Patient should be encouraged to move the shoulder and some hot fomentation of short wave diathermy may be advised.

Ferrum met: has cracking in joints, particularly in the shoulder, has an irresistible desire to bend the arm, with intense pain. Sudden cramps or tearing pain in the limbs. Rheumatic symptoms, especially of the left shoulder.

Thiosenaminum: it is useful in torn ligaments, especially in the shoulder.

Rhus toxicodendron: the joint is hot and painful swelling. The pains are tearing, and spreads over a large surface of the nape of the neck, better by motion. Limbs get stiff and paralysed. Worse after midnight, blows, jar, riding, ice-cold drinks.

Ruta: is one of the chief remedies for injured joints, tendons, bruised bones. Cracking of joints, worse walking in the open air. Tendons are sore aching pain. Worse from over-exertion injury.

Sanguinaria: rheumatism of the right shoulder. Cutting pain or stiffness in the right deltoid, worse on raising and turning arm. Pain is worse at night.

6. ***A child or a young adult complains of acute pain and often swelling in several joints. As the inflammation subsides in these joints others are affected. The patient has high temperature and there may be cardiac involvement — endocarditis. The condition is ACUTE RHEUMATISM (Acute Rheumatic Fever).***

There is usually a history of tonsillitis due to (haemolytic streptococcus) infection a week or two previous to the present complaint. The attack of acute rheumatism comes on with fever and joint pains appear within 24 hours. The usual accompaniment of fever present. The joint pains are wandering and without suppuration. One by one the joints get affected with the resolution of swelling and pain of the previous joint. The joints are acutely painful on the slightest movement, warm and tender to touch and more likely to show effusion in adults. Cardiac involvement is the most important; is less amenable to treatment and the permanent damage sets in. In children, mitral endocarditis sets in.

Aconite, Belladonna, Bryonia, Arsenic alb, Rhus tox: are those remedies which are normally indicated at the onset of the fever. If prescribed in time, chances are that the condition can be aborted.

After the acute phase of temperature is over, the pains in the limbs and joints are experienced by the patient.

Colchicum: it affect markedly muscles, fibrous tissue, serous membrane, small joints, with stitching pains in the muscles, periosteum and the joints. These shift rapidly and the swellings are very minimal. Tingling, crawling. Pains are digging, drawing worse by mental exertion and emotions, slightest touch and vibrations. There is anxiety in the region of the heart, oppression, better on walking. The pains are worse in the evening and warm weather. Joints become stiff and feverish, shifting rheumatism.

Kalmia latifolia: it has prominent action on the heart. The pains are neuralgic, and tingling numbness, trembling and paralytic weakness. Deltoid rheumatism is common, fluttering heart with anxiety. Pains along the ulnar nerve, goes into third or fourth finger. The joints are red hot, tingling and numbness of the left arm. Neuralgia of the right side, wandering rheumatic pains, which travel from above downwards, tumultuous action of the heart and slow pulse.

7. ***A woman complains of stiffness and later pain and swelling in the joints of the fingers. And later there is affection of the larger joints. This condition progresses and is associated with constitutional symptoms and some pyrexia. The condition is probably RHEUMATOID ARTHRITIS.***

Rheumatoid arthritis (RA) is a chronic multi-systemic disease of unknown etiology. The characteristic expression of RA is persistent inflammatory synovitis, usually affecting the peripheral joints in symmetric distribution. But there is a possibility of variety of systemic manifestations.

Rheumatoid Arthritis usually presents with insidious onset of pain and stiffness, in the small joints of the hands and feet which eventually lead to characteristic bilateral symmetrical peripheral polyarthritis.

These pains are worse in the morning on waking up, and may improve with activity. Often there are pains in the night and sleep gets disturbed. The morning stiffness often lasts for long hours. Fatigue and general malaise are common. There are also non-articular symptoms present like swelling, caused by effusion, warmth, tenderness on pressure or movement. Deformities occur in the later stages of the disease.

Rheumatoid Arthritis is a multi-miasmatic disorder and all these miasmatic expression can follow one after the other or can be present at one time. Psoric inflammatory stage, proliferative sycotic phase, and destructive tubercular and syphilitic phase need to be treated at their phases in a case.

Treatment will depend upon the constitution and the phase in which one receives the case.

Calcarea carb: it is an anti-psoric constitutional remedy. Persons of scrofulous type, who take cold easily. Tendency to grow fat. Disorders caused by working in water. In the back there is pain as if sprained, can scarcely rise from overlifting. Vertebrae feel loose, painful on pressure. Rheumatism of the lumbar region with weakness in the small of the back. Neck stiff and rigid. Faulty development of bones. Calcarea has cold clamy feet as if wet stockings are on, with lot of growing pains. Joints as if sprained. Rheumatoid pain as after exposure to cold. The joints look deformed, especially the knee. Arthritic nodosities, cold, sour, swelling, perspiration, burning of soles of feet are some of the charcteristics. While taking the history for RA apart from the local symptoms of the pains in the joint these characteristic qualities will be considered.

Calcarea fluoricum: there are bony growths, exostosis, and deformities of bones. Cracking in joints and easy joint dislocation, and synovial swellings. Chronic synovitis of the knee joint. Joints are worse at the beginning of the movement. Worse with the cold weather but always better in warmth. There is crepitation of joints from lack of synovial fluid. Piercing, darting, grinding pains in all joints. Cramps in muscles of legs.

Apis mel: it forms serous inflammation with effusion, extreme sensitive to touch, great burning and stinging in the affected parts — worse from heat in any form. Rheumatic pains in the back. Stiffness in the back of the neck. Knees are swollen, sensitive shining sore with stinging pains. Any joint that is affected looks puffy and red, shining and sensitive to touch.

Formica rufa: causes many rheumatic and gouty pains the pains — which appear suddenly and dart from place to place. Rheumatism comes on suddenly, with restlessness. Muscles feel torn from their attachment. Stiffness and contracture of joints.

Guaiacum: tearing and stinging in the limbs. Contractions of the affected parts. Marked stiffness of the affected limb. Joints are swollen, puffy and hot. Cannot tolerate pressure or heat.

Colchicum: it is a cold damp weather remedy especially in spring and autumn. It acts on the fibrous tissue, on the periosteum, and synovial membranes of joints, especially the small joints. It does not tend to suppuration. The joints are swollen and puffy, sensitive to touch or jars. Large joints are intensely red and hot, small joints are swollen numb and stiff. Pains go from left to right. Stitches in the right shoulder.

Kali iodatum: useful in chronic periosteal rheumatism of syphilitic origin. The condition is aggravated at night and lying on painful side. Jerking of tendons, contractions, tendons are hard and stiff, drawn tightly to palms, chilliness predominates.

Pulsatilla: wandering pains shift rapidly from place to place, and ever-changing symptoms. Caused by getting wet in the rains or water and protracted hot weather.

8. ***A middle-aged or elderly patient complains of progressive pain in one of the several joints; stiffness and grating are felt on movement but there are no constitutional symptoms. The disease is likely to be OSTEOARTHRITIS.***

Osteoarthritis (OA) is degenerative joint disease. No predisposing factor is apparent. Pain is typically in the knees, hips or hands, they are worse in the evenings and aggravated by movement, relieved by rest. Initially the pains are intermittent. Morning stiffness lasting up to half an hour or so and stiffness after sitting.

Characteristic swelling hard and bony, sometimes associated with effusion. Crepitus on movements. Signs of inflammation, warmth in the knee, and erythema in the small joints of the hand. Limitations of the movement follow with wasting of muscles around the affected joint.

Bryonia alba: joints are painful red, swollen and hot, with stitches and tearing worse on least movement. Every spot is painful on pressure. Pains better by lying down and the same side of pain. Knees totter and bend under him while walking. Knee is stiff and painful. The muscles are sore and painful. Mucus membranes are dry and serous membranes are inflamed.

The modalities are characteristic. Better on lying on the painful side, by pressure, rest and cold things. Better from bandaging. Better by drawing knees up. Irritability of mind and tissues runs through the remedy. Dropsical swelling of the leg, sensitive to touch, joints are stiff and red, swollen, stitching pains with the slightest touch.

Kali carb: Weakness is caused by all the salts of potassium, but Kali carb has these symptoms pronounced. There is weakness of the muscles of the heart, back of the limbs, including the weakness of the intellect. Fibrous tissues, ligaments of joints of uterus, of lumbar back are particularly affected. Producing relaxation, joints give way, back feels as if broken, and the patient feels compelled to lie down or lean on something. Sharp stitching pains, stabbing or catching pains are felt in various parts of the body joints, chest, muscles, head, lying on affected side. Back is stiff, and paralytic feeling, with burning in spine. Lower back feels weak. Pain in the buttocks extends to thighs, even to the knees.

Rhus tox: it affects the fibrous tissues, markedly joints, tendons, sheaths etc., producing pain and stiffness. It causes stiffness of the muscles and joints. He is always better in changing position. The ailments are from strain, over-lifting and getting wet while perspiring. The pains are tearing, shooting, and stitching, worse at night and cannot rest in any one position — therefore restless. Rheumatic pains are in damp cold weather. Better by heat and hot bath, elevating the feet.

Ruta: bursitis cracking in joints, worse on walking in open air. Pains and stiffness in the fingers and wrist. Knees give way while ascending and going down. Tendons are sore. Aching pain in the Achilles.

Kalmia lat: the pains of Kalmia are neuralgic. It is a rheumatic remedy. Pains shift rapidly, shooting outwards along the nerve. Deltoid rheumatism, especially at night. Pains from hip to knees. Kalmia pains travel from above downwards. Pains are worse from motion (Bry).

Phytolacca: rheumatic pains worse in the morning, mostly in the shoulders, with stiffness, causing difficulty in raising the arm. Pains fly like electric shock — shooting lancinating and shifting rapidly. Sharp cutting in the hips, legs are drawn up and cannot touch the ground. Aching of heels, relieved by elevating feet.

Hot painful swelling of the joints. Soreness of the condyles of the bone, limbs are stiff and paralysed. Intolerance to cold fresh air. Rheumatoid pains develop about the joints, painful stiffness in the back.

Ledum palustre: it affects the fibrous tissue of small joints — ankles, tendons, heels, and skin. Rheumatism begins in the lower limbs and spreads upward, cramps over the hip joint, cracking of joints, worse on warmth of bed, heels are sore, can hardly step on them. Easy spraining of ankles and feet, tendon. Ankles are swollen and tender after injury, better by application of ice.

Manganum aceticum: it has special affinity for periosteum of shin bones, joints, ankles and lower limbs. Inflammation of bones with nightly digging pains, growing pains and weak ankles. General soreness and aching, every part of the body feels sore when touched. It has chronic arthritis, with infiltrated glistening joints. Suppuration of the skin around the joints. Shiny and red swelling of the joints, knee pain and itching, burning spots about the joint.

OAN (Osteoarthritic nosode): it is made from the synovial liquid of arthritic joints. Pains are aggravated by the first movement, at night, better by prolonged movement. Worse right side. Pains are more marked in the Achilles tendon.

9. ***Patient, usually a tired housewife who has been gaining weight and whose spine is assuming faulty posture, experiences dull nagging pain in the lumbo-sacral area which aggravates after sitting in a chair in a flexed position, or while stretching the back with knees straight, especially after lifting a heavy weight. The condition is LOW BACK PAIN or LUMBAGO.***

One should differentiate this condition from more frequently presented condition which sets in with sudden crippling pain, often spreading into one or both sciatic nerve, called **Intervertebral Disc Lesion**, and **Osteoarthritis of the lumbar spine**, and **Ankylosing Spondylitis**.

In fact it will be worth while to refer to a repertory for these conditions since there are so many modifying symptoms which need to be considered. But most common remedies indicated will be discussed:

Rhus Tox: according to Hahnemann, Rhus tox is is the most efficacious and a specific remedy for frequently fatal effects of over-lifting, inordinate exertions of muscles and contusions. His observation led to the most important symptom — bruised and sprain-like and stiffness in the back. There is stiff neck with painful tension when moving. Pain and stiffness in the small of the back, better motion when lying on something hard, worse while sitting. The backache is constrictive, better on hard pressure or bending backwards. Rhus affects fibrous tissues — markedly joints, tendons, sheaths, producing pain and stiffness. Motion limbers up the Rhus patient and he, therefore, feels better for a time from change of position. Cold damp season is worse.

Tellurium: has restlessness and pains all over the body, very sensitive back. Afraid cannot bear to be touched on sensitive areas. Sacral and sciatic pains. Weak feeling in the back, pressing aches in the scapula, numbness in the nape and occiput. Pain from the last cervical to the fifth dorsal vertebra, very sensitive to pressure and touch. Sensitive spinal column on coughing and sneezing, straining. The neck pain spreads into shoulder, and between the scapula. Lumbar pain spreads to the right thigh, ameliorated by walking.

Sepia: there is weakness in the small of the back when walking, usually associated with uterine complaints. Collar feels tight, coldness between the shoulders, sudden pain in the back as if struck by hammer, worse on stooping, and kneeling. Back pain is better by belching, by pressing back against something. Hard stiffness of limbs; worse after sleep.

Cimicifuga: The pain across the pelvis from hip to hip. Menses are with severe backache, more the flow more the pain. Useful in rheumatic persons, Plump, delicate, sensitive, nervous, chilly, women who complain of aching pain in the back, neck, here and there. Rhematic pains in the muscles of back and neck. Stiffness and contractions in neck and back. Pain in the neck is worse sensitive and worse on pressure, which causes nausea. Pain in the lumbar and sacral regions, down thighs and through hips, crick in the back.

Aesculus: There is a characteristic backache that incapacitates the patient and makes him useless for any work. Backache of sacrum and hips, worse on walking or stooping. Pains are lightening. Back feels weak. He has to make repeated efforts to rise from sitting position. Pains are so severe that it makes almost impossible to walk.

10. ***Patient complains of dull aching or burning pain in the occipital area or in the lower neck or in the arm, associated with paraesthesiae. The condition is CERVICAL OSTEOARTHRITIS or SPONDYLOSIS.***

It is usually due to postero-lateral disc protrusion and, sometimes, to changes in the articular surfaces. The result is narrowing of the intervertebral foramina by osteophytes. Between cervical C-3 -7, specially in the C5 and C6-7 area. Initially there is complaint of stiffness, and limitation of movement. Gradually this becomes more aggravated and causes compression of the cervical nerve roots.

Rhus Toxicodendron: rheumatic pains spread over a large area of the surface of the neck, better by motion. Soreness of the condyles of the bone, limbs become stiff and paralysed. Cannot tolerate fresh cold air. After overwork there is pain in the limbs. Pains travel along the ulnar nerve. Loss of power in the hands and forearm with crawling sensation in the tips of the fingers.

Lachnantes tinctoria: there is stiff neck and the head is drawn to one side, with rheumatism of the neck, the pain is as if dislocated. Tearing from the shoulder, extending to finger joint, thumb and index finger feel as if sprained.

Radium bromatum: sharp pains in the shoulder, arms, hand, fingers. Neck feels very hard and brittle and feels as if they would break on moving. Pain and lameness in the cervical vertebrae, worse on dropping head forward, better on standing or sitting erect.

Paris quadrifolia: there is weight and weariness in the nape of the neck. Violent pain in both sides of the neck, extending down to fingers; worse on mental exertion. Neuralgia beginning in the left intercostal region and extending to the left arm. Arms become stiff, fingers clenched, fingers feel numb, and everything feels rough. It is a left-sided remedy but coldness is in the right side of the body while the left side is natural and hot.

In all these cases of lumbar spine spondylosis, more than the remedies physiotheraphy will be very useful. A competent physiotherapist can give good and appropriate exercises so that the condition can be greatly eased quickly.

9 GERIATRIC MANAGEMENT (Diseases of the elderly)

- Atrophy of the Skin
- Angina Pectoris
- Enlargement of Prostate Gland
- Delayed Union of Fracture
- Deafness

"oh love playthings well as a child,
to lead an adventurous and honourable youth,
and to settle when the time arrives into a green and smiling age,
is to be a good artist in life."

R. L. Stevenson.

The process of ageing is common to all animals and its scientific study is known as gerentology (Greek *geron*, an old man).

While most men and women may be judged as good 'artists in life,' there are some who are unfortunate in not finding an old age green and smiling. As life advances both physical and psychological disorders become more common and severe. Therefore difficulties in adjusting to social environment increase.

Geriatrics is that branch of medicine devoted to the problem of old age and its sociological, pathological, psychological and clinical aspects.

The concept of life-span is that there is a limit beyond which an individual cannot survive. The life machine cannot go on forever and it has to stop clicking sometime. It was a common belief that man survives to about 70 years of life. But this life-span has now increased. Average life-span is about 65 for males and 60 for females in India. In the developed countries like U.K., U.S.A, Japan the figures are about 75 for males and 70 for females. This increase is because of many changes having taken place in the development of medicine, awareness of hygiene, sanitation, improvement in nutrition. But this increase in life-span has created different problems for these elderly persons.

Ageing can be described as progressive constriction of homeostatic reserve of every organ system. This decline is often called homeostenosis. This homeostenosis is evident by third decade of life which is gradual and progressive. Although the rate of this progressive decline is different in speed and extent. The decline of each organ system takes place independently of changes in the other system. This change is influenced by diet, environment, personal habits as well as genetic factors.

— There is no stereotype ageing. Individuals become dissimilar as they age.

— An abrupt decline in any system or function is always due to disease and not due to ageing.

— Normal ageing can be hastened by risk factor like smoking, blood pressure and sedentary life-style etc.

— Irrespective of disease or not, healthy ageing homeostatic reserve causes no symptoms and imposes few restrictions on the daily activity regardless of age say around 70 to 80 years.

In an elderly an organ or system is affected which has already been affected physiologically or pathologically earlier. Because of these organ changes this system behaves differently from system or organ in an young. The disease presentation can be atypical in an elderly. For example, elderly with hypothyroidism may present signs of goiter, tremors and exophthalmos and there may be atrial fibrillation, confusion, depression, syncope, and weakness. Similarly, because the weakest link is the brain, limited number of prominent symptoms will present — acute confusion, incontinence, falling etc. no matter what is the underlying disease. Because of their impaired physiological reserve, older patients often present at an early stage of the disease. For example patient may come with retention of urine with mild prostate enlargement, mild hyperthyroidism may precipitate heart failure or coma by mild glucose intolerance. A small improvement in one area may dramatically change the course to betterment quickly.

Many findings that are abnormal in younger age group are relatively common in elderly — premature ventricular contractions, bacteriuria, low bone mineral density, impaired glucose tolerance. However all the symptoms may not be dismissed as old-age symptoms, but must be thoroughly investigated. Symptoms in elderly may be due to various causes. Older patients suffer the consequences of the disease, ***treatment and preventive management is more effective***.

Loss of hair pigment is because of loss of melanocytes, their looks become old because of changes in the skin, and wrinkles are formed because of atrophy of subcutaneous fat.

There is an increase in the hypersensitivity and, hence, there is increase in the drug reaction in elderly people.

It is necessary to emphasize here that most old people are physically and mentally independent and can live on their own resources. Even when they become dependent they still can manage with family and neighbourly support till their last illness.

Although great social changes have taken place in the Western world over the last two decades but here in India the traditional family ties have still remained strong.

Some erosion is seen in the cities and urban areas. That is mainly because of the hectic life, industrial revolution, shortage of living space and high cost of living. In the past extended family thrived in teeming life. Today the extended family is less important and people prefer nucleus or primary family composed of father, mother and their offspring. This might have happened due to sheer necessity but then elder couple who had the fortune of the children and grand-children around suddenly find themselves cut off and start finding themselves lonely — physically and psychologically. Very often adjustment becomes a very difficult task even after counselling because it is very difficult for a old person to change his habits cultivated over the years so fast because their 'ego' comes in the way. Psychologically, widow is a greater sufferer because she finds it difficult to adjust with another younger woman in the house who is at the helm of affairs.

Management of these problems should start much in advance. 'Prevention is better than cure'. Pre-retirement counselling should be organized. This will make the person aware of the problems that he may face and help him prepare to face them. The subjects should deal with (1) Health education — the role of diet, regular exercise and maintenance of social life. (2) Financial implication of retiral life so that he knows what will be his income and what would be his investments and how he can mobilize resources in case of any emergencies. (3) Services available for old people — who are still healthy and can put in some work, and (4) Use of leisure time such as hobbies, handicrafts, and voluntary work. This will help these people psychologically and they will not feel the pinch of loneliness.

Approach to the therapeutic management of the case is like any other case. That has already been explained earlier. Totality of case is important. But in clinical practice few homoeopathic remedies which have the affinity to such cases may be kept in mind.

Management of the old age problems can be handled in two ways. One is by providing medical treatment for the conditions presented by the patient. And second is by counselling the patient and the persons around the patient.

One will appreciate that there can be no remedies that can be sited. In fact, in no disorder there can be set remedies which can be spelled out. All will depend on the totality of the symptoms arrived at after the analysis of the case history. However we have certain remedies in our materia medica which promise good results. In these circumstances, judicious use of these remedies along with the remedy arrived after the totality picture can give desired results.

It is observed that ageing is accompanied by physiological decline, diminishing power of adaptation and increased vulnerability to stress, increase in diseases. They also show diminished power to survive trauma, and to resist and overcome infection. Stress causes profound effect on the ageing body, and that too takes a long time to restore the normal internal environment.

Skin has characteristic changes in the aged, it becomes atrophied and loses elasticity and develops wrinkles.

Most people develop atherosclerosis at an early age and this condition becomes severe with advanced age, although the process is very slow and gradual and it may not reach clinical significance. The condition increases in severity with age and affects other vessels, e.g coronary and cerebral arteries. Mental confusion is the result of severe atherosclerotic changes in the cerebral arteries resulting in cerebral ischaemia. Similar changes may occur in the coronary arteries causing coronary ischaemia.

Old people sometimes exhibit retardation of healing process, for example fracture may not heal easily. In bone there is decrease in the osteoid matrix, osteoporosis that tends to develop and the bones break easily in old people than in young people, mainly because of decreased estrogen at the time of menopause, which causes changes in reproductive tissues and marked changes in the bone metabolism that leads to osteoporosis with other risk factors. There is a progressive decline in testosterone levels in men with ageing. There is atrophy of the gonads, both in older men and women.

The aged brain takes longer to appreciate a stimulus to identify its nature and to select the most appropriate response.

There is a failure of short term retention of data in the aged because of easy distraction of attention from the problem under consideration. Similarly there is difficulty in recalling information. The speed of movement is lost in the elderly but is compensated by increased accuracy.

Age-associated changes in vision and hearing may contribute to significant functional impairment in older adults. Visual acuity may decrease due to changes in the retina or neural elements.

Hearing changes occur both in peripheral auditory system and at the level of cerebral cortex.

1. ***An elderly person complains of terrible itching, with wrinkles on his skin, and the skin shows loss of elasticity. The condition is ATROPHY OF THE SKIN.***

This is a very common condition of the skin in the aged unless it is accompanied by any infection. The natural process of degeneration of the skin with the age has set in and one cannot stop this process. Only thing one can do is to retard this process or delay the changes and reduce the unpleasant symptoms accompanying the process. The general health of the patient will decide the prognosis.

Croton Tiglium: it produces erythema, erysipelas, eczema, herpes pustules. There is plenty of itching. But the patient cannot bear to scratch very hard as it hurts, a very light rubbing allays the itching. Otorrhoea when there is lot of itching.

Secale cornutum: the skin is shrivelled, numb, dusky blue tinge, cold, dry, wrinkled worse over the affected parts. Twitching and quivering in the skin,with formication under the skin. Burning sensation better by cold, wants parts uncovered. Skin cold to touch, yet the covering is not tolerated. Slight wounds continue to bleed.

Sepia: the skin is delicate, the least injury tends to ulcerate. Itching often changes to burning when scratched. Soreness of the skin on bends of the knee. Ringworm-like eruption on the face and on different parts of the body every spring. Better in warm room. Desperate itching especially when there is eruption on the genitals and anus.

Alumina: dry skin with inability to perspire. Dry and cracked skin. Intolerable itching when getting warm in bed, must scratch until it bleeds. All the skin symptoms get aggravated in winter, full and new moon.

There are many other drugs which are indicated in this type of skin of the elderly, and one should remember to consider entire drug as a whole.

2. *An elderly person complains of dyspnoea, weak and rapid pulse, heart failure is threatened with slightest exertion either because of valvular disease or anaemia. It is a case of ANGINA PECTORIS, or MYOCARDITIS or CARDIAC DILATATION.*

Crataegus oxyacantha: it is nearest approach to heart tonic and is not the heart poison as digitalis. It is a heart tonic, and does not produce any cumulative effect. It is a sedative in cross, irritable patients with cardiac symptoms. The patient suddenly becomes weak and exhausted with high blood pressure. Creatagus 5 drop doses of mother tincture is a dose that should be administered five times daily for a long period.

Digitalis: least movement causes violent palpitation, and a sudden sensation as if heart stood still. Palpitation from depression from grief. Heart is tired after sprains. Hypertrophy with dilatation, irregular heart, especially with mitral valve disease. The greatest indication is failure of compensation, specially when auricular fibrillation has set in. Great weakness and sinking of strength, faintness and coldness of skin and irregular respiration, cardiac irritability.

Cactus grandiflorus: chief action is around the heart and the circulation. Many complaints are associated with heart disorders. Atheromatous arteries, and weak heart. Cactus produces characteristic constriction feeling as from an iron band. Body feels tight or wrapped. Hot gushing in the chest. Fainting, pulseless, panting, and prostration, low blood pressure from weakness of the heart. Congestion and irregular distribution of blood. Palpitation is worse on lying on left side. Pulsation increases on holding the breath. Endocarditis, with mitral insufficiency together with rapid and violent action.

3. *An elderly patient complains of frequency of urination, usually noted as night difficulty or delay in initiating urination with variability and reduced force of the urinary stream, and post-void dribbling. The condition is BENIGN ENLARGEMENT OF PROSTATE GLAND.*

Conium maculatum: Conium corresponds to elderly people. Old feeble men, old maids and bachelors with strong sedentary habits and those who are easily intoxicated by stimulants. Scrofulous constitution and glandular enlargement. Difficulty of passing urine in the beginning even when standing, and then it flows freely. Interrupted urination stops and starts. Better standing, dribbling in old men. Cutting and burning after urination. Testicles are hard and enlarged. Prostatitis, dribbling of prostatic fluid. Worse stools, emotions. With decreased power has increased desire. Often without any erection.

Clematis erecta: tingling in urethra lasting some time after urination. Frequent scanty urination, burning in urethra during urination and last drop causes violent burning. Urine stops and starts, or dribbles after urination.

Staphysagria: enlarged prostate with haemorrhoids, and pain extends from anus to urethra. Pain running from anus, along urethra, inflamed testicles with shooting and drawing in the cords, stitching towards groin and testicles.

Sabal serrulata: enlargement of prostate. Constant desire to pass urine at night, paresis of the bladder sphincter, incontinence from any exertion. Like lifting, laughing. Cystitis from prostate enlargement. Impotence and loss of sexual power, sex is painful at the time of emission.

Selenium: frequent urination with urgent need to urinate, involuntary dribbling when walking. Dribbling of urine after urination and after stool. Prostatitis with dribbling of prostatic fluid, irritability after sex. but there is loss of sexual power. Lascivious but impotent. Easy loss of semen during coitus, with feeble erection.

4. ***An elderly person who had a fall more than six weeks ago complains that the repeat X-ray of the fracture site shows that the fracture has not healed. The condition is DELAYED UNION OF FRACTURE.***

This delay is because of slow formation of callous in the bone at the site of the fracture. This can happen in the brittle bones.

Calcarea phos: Calcarea phos affects the nutrition of the bones and glands. Bones become soft, thin and brittle and Cal phos promotes the ossification of the bones in the non-union of fractures. In any case there must be other symptoms of Cal phos. in general.

Symphytum Officinale: Symphytum is the bone remedy. Useful in injuries to bones, cartilage and periosteum. Painful old injuries fractures and broken bones. Pricking and stitching pains remaining after wound is healed. Non-union of fractures with deficient callus. Arthralgia of joints. External application disposes the swelling due to injury or other growths. Bruises, sprains and inflammation of bones facilitated its quick healing.

Silicea: Useful in diseases of bones and cartilages, decay and necrosis, softening of bones. Silica can stimulate the organism to reabsorb fibrotic conditions, and scar tissue.

5. ***An elderly person complains of gradual loss of hearing. This is DEAFNESS due to otosclerosis.***

One should evaluate his loss of hearing. Try and find out whether there are any associated complaints. Associated complaints are usually tinnitus, vertigo, difficulty in balancing, earache, otorrhoea, and aural fullness. And carefully reconstruct the history of evolution of the hearing deficit. Gradual deficit in hearing is common with oto sclerosis.

Graphites: There is hardness of hearing, but hears better in noise. Hissing in the ears. Tinnitus. There is sudden detonation like report of a gun in the ear. Dryness in the inner ear. Thin white scaly membrane covering the eardrum. Sensation as if air is filled with water. Cracking in the ears while eating.

Pulsatilla: Hearing is difficult, as if the ear was stuffed. Deafness as if the ear was stoppped. Can hear better in warm room and a moving car. Otorrhoea, discharge of pus, of blood thick yellow humor offensive after exanthema.

China sulph: Violent ringing, buzzing in the ears. Deafness with tinnitus, Usually the tinnitus in the left ear and there is deafness. Associated with this, at times, there is violent headache. Useful in Meniere's disease.

Hepar sulph: Whizzing and throbbing in the ear, with hardness of hearing. Deafness is from eustachian catarrh after scarlet fever. Painful otitis media, and ears are sensitive to touch.

As said earlier there can be no set disorders in old age. A that is found often is the continuation of diseases originated in the younger age which depends on the heredity, exposure to various environments, modification of susceptibilities. These coupled with the reduced resistance of old age, natural changes in the metabolism present the disease picture.

The pathogenesis of certain homoeopathic remedies point to multiple actions in these elderly and can cover many old age conditions. Those curable can be cured but those which are incurable are paliated so that the patient is comfortable. Few of such remedies are:

Ambra grisea: is temperamentally a nervous personality. Insomnia is a characteristic complaint particularly arising from worries and anxiety. Although very tired he just can't sleep. Another important factor is loss of memory. Forgetful and cannot remember the simplest fact. Because of defective nervous system the drug responses also get altered. Being a nosode it can be used as an intercurrent remedy to correct the altered drug response.

Conium maculatum: is known remedy for the disorders of the old people. These old people have had some exhaustive diseases and Conium tends to correct this exhaustion. In cardiovascular system action of the heart is weak, with irregular pulse, in various glands of the body there is stony hard mass. In breast fibroadenoma, or benign mastitis after injury, or orchitis in testes, in prostate there is stop and flow situation in the stream of the urine, and the flow is better standing, an early prostatitis, in the nervous system there is due to cerebral anaemia, vertigo on turning the head when in bed.

Baryta Carb: it is known for the action on both extremities of life. It is more suited to old age when there are mental symptoms. There is a peculiar aversion to strangers. There are some elderly people who do not like the approach of an unfamiliar face and have fear of the presence of other. They get easily angered. Following an acute attack of apoplexy they tend to develop paralysis. They develop loss of memory. In old people chest is weak and they suddenly develop a chill and catarrh, sensation of smoke in the chest causing dyspnoea. And this aggravation takes place in wet and warm weather.

Senega: it has its action on the mucous membrane causing catarrhal symptoms especially of respiratory tract, bladder and eyes. Asthmatic bronchitis often with emphysema, or chronic nephritis. Opacities of vitreous humour.

Lachesis: its use is well-known to all homoeopaths. It's use in the menopausal condition in the females is important, provided the patient has aggravation from heat and in the evening or after sleep.There is great physical and mental tension. High blood pressure and manic depressions are common.

For general muscular weakness:

Gelsemium: there is loss of power of muscular control, excessive trembling, weakness of all the limbs. Cramps in the wrist, professional neurosis, writer's cramp, weak limbs while climbing with tottering gait, great fatigue after slight exercise. Staggering as if intoxicated when trying to move, with dizziness and blurred vision.

Phosphoric acid: there is weakness with great debility, Pain in the bones as if scraped. Tearing pains in the joints bones and the periosteum. Prostatorrhoea even when passing a soft stool. Sleepy by day, hot and wakeful by night, but short sleep rests him. In diabetes there is history of sexual excess or of severe mental strain. The urine while passing is clear but turns white on standing.

Causticum : Paralysis of single parts, trembling of hands, cannot lift hand, cannot walk without suffering. Unsteady walking and easily falling with weak ankles. Pains like electric shock, restless in the limbs. Prostatitis and frequent urethritis, and cannot retain urine. Warts are notable features in the hands.

For osteoarthritis and rheumatoid arthritis or disc prolapse which are particularly troublesome in the old age **Bryonia, Rhustox, Manganum aceticum, Formic acid, Tellurium** should be remembered.

There can be no limit to this list. Since there is no specific remedy for one single condition we have to depend on the totality.

Along with the medication what is equally important is counselling. Loneliness is one of the most important psychological block that can cause a condition or prolong a condition, in spite of the right treatment. Foresaken, unwanted feeling, feeling of neglect in the family can cause a lot of depressive condition and sometimes the will to live is lost. With right type of counselling to the patient and the relatives intercurrent remedies like Ignatia, Phosphoric acid, Staphysagria, Natrum mur, Aurum met can help. As said earlier the patient must find a vocation to keep himself busy, take up painting, reading or working in social organizations. In fact, change of attitude is necessary in both the patient as well as the relatives around. The patient must learn to adjust to the changed times. If this is accepted then the indicated remedies will work to get the desired result.

10 DISORDERS OF ENDOCRINES AND METABOLISM

- Simple Goitre
- Hyperthyroidism
- Hypothyroidism
- Gout
- Diabetes Mellitus

Our constitutional remedies possess great potentiality in maintaining good health, when prescribed on the basic principle of 'law of similars'. We should utilize this property through the potentized remedies to correct the erring constitutional processes by bringing balance in the endocrinal secretions. Imbalance in the production of these endocrines cause various disorders which show through various signs and symptoms. The clusters of these signs and symptoms are recognized in clinical practice by various syndromes depending on the increase or the decrease of production of these secretions. In practice we often meet situations when there is no alternative than external substitution of these hormones. Recovery through this process is, no doubt, very quickly achieved but it may not be permanent in nature and the therapy will be required almost lifelong.

There are many known syndromes concerning reproduction and Sex, Growth, Thyroid, Gluco-corticoid, Endocrinology of Hypertension control etc. But we shall consider here only those conditions which present often for treatment to a homoeopathic physician. On evaluation we need to decide their therapy. Very many cures have shown the efficacy of this treatment.

Our polychrest remedies have sufficient depth to influence the glandular conditions. If we closely study these polychrests they belong to the same chemical base that our body is made up of such as Sulphur, Phosphorus, Silicea, Potassium (Kali), Sodium (Natrum) or Magnesium and Carbon.

1. ***A female patient, usually in her teens, presents with an enlargement of the thyroid gland but does not present with any uncomfortable symptoms warranting a treatment except that it is unsightly. The condition is SIMPLE GOITRE.***

Simple goitre is either endemic or sporadic or diffuse or nodular. Most of these simple goitres are due to dietary insufficiency of iodine. These are presented by people living in isolated villages and often in high mountains, for example Nepal. These people migrate in search for jobs. Change of diet and addition of iodized salt in their food greatly improves the condition. Most of the time no treatment is required. However it is necessary to inquire into food habits of the patient and if any objectionable food being taken in large quantities is detectable then that item of food may be eliminated.

Constitutional remedies like Calcarea, Natrum muriaticum, Iodium and Spongia closely resemble the pathogenesis of the simple goitre.

During puberty and pregnancy goitre associated with euthyroidism rarely requires intervention. Patient should be reassured that that there will be spontaneous resolution.

Very often Goitre is noticed as cosmetic defect. The majority of them are painless, but can produce dysphagia and difficulty in breathing implying oesophageal or tracheal compression. Clinical thyroid status of these patients must be determined.

2. ***A patient tall for her age and sex, reports with moderately enlarged soft and highly vascular thyroid gland with a conspicuous lobular structure : complains that the growth has been slowly developing : there is general heat and feels feverish, the appetite is increased but not sufficient to compensate the increase in energy expenditure, and hence patient complains of loss of weight, there is palpitation and breathlessness on exertion, resting pulse rate is raised often over 100/min., raised systolic pressure, and peripheral vasodilation, cardiac arrhythmia, great anxiety with fine tremors to the hands, diarrhoea, irregular menstruation. The condition is HYPERTHYROIDISM.***

This is a clinical condition resulting from increased levels of free T4 and or T3, usually because of the disorder of the Thyroid gland but can also be induced by administration of excessive amounts of thyroidal hormones.

Clinical features of hyperthyroidism are seen through many systems. There is loss of weight although appetite is greatly increased. Behavioural change and increased irritability, and restlessness. There is heat intolerance, breathlessness, palpitation, loss of libido etc.

No treatment should be instituted without biochemical confirmation. TSH is suppressed, and a normal TSH usually excludes the diagnosis.

If one studies the pathogenesis of Iodides of Kalium, Baryta, Natrum, Magnesium, Spongia, Bromium one will find a close resemblance to the pathogenesis of hyperthyroidism.

Kali iod: has strong action on the tumours of glands, tumours of the breast . Kali iod craves open air and motion. Patient has rheumatic, gouty diathesis. Pains are characteristic — crushing, stitching and sharp pains. Discharges are watery and foul. There is loss of weight. There is diffused sensitiveness over the affected parts. Goitre is sensitive to touch.

Baryta iod: has been used in enlarge thyroid, enlarged breasts with tumours.

Spongia: has usually these tumours which develop after blows or injury. Usually the lower potencies are useful, use.30c. : action on the lymphatic and glandular system. . The testes and the thyroid are indurated. The blood , heart and the veins are involved and with the protruding eyes a perfect picture of exophthalmic expression.

Thyroidinum: an important sarcode is of great use in the cases of thyroid — both in its excessive state or reduced state. This Thyroidinum is now better known as Iodothyrine. It is prepared from the dried thyroid gland of a sheep. It is interesting that Thyroidinum 3x is often found useful in hypothyroidism and Thyroidinum 6x is useful in hyperthyroidism. While using this sarcode remember it will have all the signs and symptoms of the disease, one will only have to match the modalities for its proper use.

Iodum: has enlargement of glands, testes, thyroid, breast, mesenteric etc. They first get swollen, and then begin to dwindle. There is a rapid metabolism, emaciation, weight loss, and debility causing perspiration on slightest exertion. Hot patient. Ravenous appetite, yet emaciating. Goitre is hard and has sense of constriction, impending deglutition.

3. ***A female patient in her middle life, with a puffy face, baggy eyelids, and with sparse hair on the head, falling of eyelids from the outer third eyebrows, swollen and oedematous swelling of the supra-clavicular region, neck, back and hands presents for treatment. This is case of HYPOTHYROIDISM.***

This is a clinical condition resulting from decreased circulating levels of T4 and/ or T3. When this hypothyroidism is of a severe degree and of long standing, it is seen as myxoedema which is characterized by deposition of mucinous material causing swelling of the skin and of subcutaneous tissue. Many complaints related to alimentary, cardiovascular and generative organs will be presented. The treatment will depend mostly on how the case is presented. In general practice we see replacement therapy is instituted by using L thyroxine as remedy of choice. The homoeopathic treatment will be mostly on the constitution and the totality of the case. The choice of remedies will fall with Bromium, Calcarea Iodide, Graphites, Kali Iodide, Natrum mur, Sepia, Spongia and Thyroidinum.

Bromium: is useful in scrofulous children, with enlarged glands. And is mostly prescribed on the general expression, swollen and indurated glands, with much anxiety, fear of ghosts and vision in the dark. Useful in sailors who come ashore and are better at seaside.

Graphites: is useful in those who have a tendency to put on weight, unhealthy fat, defective animal heat from defective oxygenation, always cold whether indoors or outdoors. Nodulated goitre choking while swallowing, worse on empty swallowing.

Kali iodatum: has glandular swellings with loss of weight.

4. ***Patient may present with a sudden acute excruciating pain in the great toe, having started the pain in the early hours of the morning, the joint is red and swollen, and very tender. This condition is GOUT.***

Gout is caused by monosodium urate monohydrate or uric acid crystals, deposition from hyperuricaemic body fluids.

There are two stages in which this disorder presents: firstly, recurrent attacks of arthritis, and secondly, when these attacks finally do not resolve they leave behind deposition of urates in and around the joints.

An acute gouty arthritis affects the metatarso-phalangeal joints of big toe initially and later feet, ankles, knees and hands, wrist, elbow. The excruciating pains are usual at night.

Gout is a disease as obstinate as it is painful. It owes its origin usually to high living, although heredity has much to do with its development.

The treatment of Gout may be divided into that of the acute paroxysm and that of the general symptoms. In the acute attacks these have been successfully used.

Colchicum: Toe joints become inflamed, dark red and hot, and intensely painful, the foot becomes oedematous; urine scanty and dark red. The smell of the food makes him sick at the stomach. Cannot tolerate any noise and external impressions.

Ledum pal: is useful after abuse of alcoholic drinks. Hot tensive swelling of the toe, foot with tearing, grinding and shooting pains, cannot bear the least covering or the warmth of the bed. Although there is oedema of the foot there is copious and frequent urine and the nodes of the frequent attacks turn very painful and sore, better by ice application.

Arinca: the pains are unbearable during the night and the bed feels too hard. The inflamed joint is shining, red, and hard. He dreads the proximity of anyone.

Bryonia: has swollen joint, tense and not very red. Feels deathly sick and has a white-coated tongue; and is unbearably cross.

Benzoic acid: usually has a very offensive urine and deposits a reddish cloudy sediment but with attack the urine becomes more or less clear, and there is tearing sensation in the joints, old nodes become painful, and the pain abates with the palpitation in the heart and ceases only when they increase.

Belladonna: has swelling, redness of the joint with excruciating, throbbing pain ,and very sensitive to touch, and are worse from hanging down of the parts, and at night these attacks are often precipitated by taking cold. When fever is present other symptoms of Belladonna will also be present.

Mag phos: has similar pains, redness and swelling but they are better with hot fomentation.

Lycopodium: will be very useful in sub-acute and chronic cases. It has a weak digestion. There is a lot of flatulence, with bloated abdomen. Aversion to bread, desire for sweets, delicacies and pastries, cannot eat oysters and onions, beans, eating them causes severe swelling of joints due to precipitation of uric acid. Prefers hot food and drink. There is frequent urging to urinate. Pain in the back starts before passing the urine and that is better after urinating. Red sand in urine offensive. Usually there is relief in joint pain after offensive loaded urine freely passes.

Causticum: has painful nodes on the joint, stiff joints and the pains are relieved by the warmth of the bed.

Graphites: has tearing in toes, the pains drives him of the bed at night, and the gastralgia is relieved by eating.

Lithium carb: has gouty constitution and uric acid diathesis. Soreness is the key-note of lithium carb. Violent sharp pains, as from red hot needles.

Diet is very important for these patients. Foods containing high purine material need to be totally avoided. Foods like cauliflowers, beans, mushrooms need to be totall discarded. Alcohol to be stopped. Fish of crustaceous origin should also be avoided.

5. ***An adult complains of gradual development of polyuria, intense thirst, with perhaps nocturia, weight loss, weakness and lassitude, pruritus, cramps in the legs, crops of boils and loss of libido. He claims that it has been happening over some period. This condition is DIABETES MELLITUS.***

Hahnemann has classified Diabetes Mellitus on the basis of his Miasmatic Theory. Present-day classification based on the WHO Classification does not differ from what Hahnemann had thought of. Hahnemann's Psoric diabetics are those who are called Pre And Potential Diabetics of modern classification of WHO. Sycotic Diabetics are those who are Non-Insulin Dependent Diabetic (NIDDM). Grouped under Tubercular or Syphilitic type are those which are Insulin dependent (IDDM) cases.

Disposition to Diabetes is determined by the hereditary characters and the individual susceptibilities in the presence of Hostile Environment.

In clinical practice we receive three categories of cases of DM, one where there is increase in blood sugar on stress and the sugar falls down when the stress is withdrawn. These are Pre and Potential Diabetics (Psoric). These patients need counselling, exercise, proper diet, and change in life-style that would keep the stress at bay. Such patients often do not need any medical regimen. In the second group of Diabetics are confirmed cases on oral hypoglycaemic agents. Here it may be necessary to determine the cause of Diabetes. It is either untreated Psoric Diabetes or may have defective pancreatic metabolism, where there is less production of Insulin or less utilization of Insulin causing disturbance in the carbohydrate metabolism. Patient should continue the oral hypoglycaemic agent that he has been taking, and observe the same rules for his exercise and diet. In addition he can be started with Homoeopathic remedy based on his totality. It is observed that with the passage of time the need for the oral hypoglycaemic agent will become less. It may be that at the end he can withdraw the hypoglycaemic drug and, finally, he may be able to do without the homoeopathic remedy also. Only exercise and diet will be his treatment. In the third group we find the patients fully dependent on insulin. It is our observation that the continuous insulin therapy causes fall in the production of bodily insulin and then cannot do without it. Homoeopathic therapy may help for some time but not all the time. Reversal of these cases may not be fully achieved.

Let us study the first group where stress is an important factor that causes this imbalance of hormones. In the chapter of Mind (Kent) there is a rubric ***"Ailments from"***: Disappointment from Love, Bad News, Despair, Emotions, Fear, Fright, Grief, Mortification, Depression, Sadness. All these factors are capable of altering the hormonal physiology in hypersensitive or hyper-reactive individual. Remedies listed under these rubrics are ***Aconite, Nat mur, Ignatia, Phosphorus, Calcarea, Sulphur*** in Bold Type and *Argentum nit, Graphites, Psorinum* etc. in italics. We all know that these are all deep acting, strong Psoric/Tubercular remedies. These drugs have action on the overall economy of the patient, and the blood examinations may show the labile nature of their blood sugar levels when under stress. Similarly, remedies like Pulsatilla, Sepia, Natrum mur, Calcarea are listed under physical stress, exertion, or pregnancy. Severe infection can also cause elevation of Blood Sugar and once the infection goes away there is fall ugar level. These remedies will act both as inter-current and constitutional remedies. ese drugs when prescribed on the basis of the totality take care of both emotional d the subsequent physical characteristics and reduce the emotional effects and the ysiological/biochemical values. These remedies ultimately help in improving your notional states and subsequent physical changes.

If these labile state of blood sugar levels are not controlled in time the condition nay proceed to produce some structural changes in the organs which may transform the whole process to sycotic state. Apart from short period of blood sugar elevation more viable changes in the system such as polyurea, intense thirst with occasional nocturia, excessive appetite with weight loss, weakness and lassitude, loss of libido. In female patients there will be pruritus vulvae, and in males balanitis will be found.

Physiognomy of sycotic patients are different from that of Psoric or Tubercular. The whole mechanism is slow and sluggish to develop or to react. Obesity is marked in these patients and the reasons for the partial failure of the biochemic mechanism is genetic trait. Any benign or malignant tumour of the pancreas can cause damage to the pancreatic function and disturb the normal mechanism.

Sycotic remedies indicated in this condition are **Thuja, Medorrhinum, Natrum sulph, Colchicum, Pulsatilla,** etc. All these are polychrest remedies and have a deep sycotic action on the human economy.

In the third group, Insulin Dependent Diabetes Mellitus, there is nearly total failure of the pancreatic metabolism and reversibility is not often possible and there is total depedence on the external Insulin. In this the symptoms of polyuria, polydipsia, and polyphagia becoming very prominent, ketoacidosis follows with nausea, vomiting and headache. This, therefore, included in the tubercular or syphilitic dimensions. Weight loss due to fluid depletion and the accelerated break-down of the fat and muscle secondary to insulin deficiency is seen.

Phosphoric acid: is suited to persons of originally strong constitution, weakened by loss of fluids, acute diseases, chagrin or succession of moral emotions, or persons of mild disposition, or children or adults who have grown rapidly with pain in the back, with profuse watery urination, more at night, sometimes the urine — though clear on passing — turns milky and is offensive. Testes are tender and swollen with weakness of sexual power.

Uranium nit.: has excessive thirst, polyuria, and dry tongue. Uranium nit in lower potency 3x and 30 gives relief faster than any other potency. There is frequent desire to urinate — large quantities of urine with pain in the kidneys and any attempt to retain this urine causes excessive pain.

Lactic acid: both lower and higher potencies are useful.

Rhus aromaticus: there is large quantity, low specific gravity urination and there is bladder atony causing incontinence. Severe pain at the beginning of urination.

A good diabetic care comprises of organized training programme involving nurse, physician and dietician.

There cannot be set diet for all diabetic patients and, therefore, the caloric requirements are tailored to the need of the individual patient.

11 DISORDERS OF THE NERVOUS SYSTEM

- Headache
- Trigeminal Neuralgia
- Nystagmus
- Migraine
- Meniere's Syndrome
- Coma
- Epileptic Seizure
- Febrile Convulsion
- Meningitis
- Sciatica
- Stroke
- Bell's Palsy
- Cervical Spondylitis
- Myesthenia Gravis
- Multiple Sclerosis

There has been a dramatic change over the last fifty years in neurological conditions seen in our routine daily practice. This has become possible because of the treatment and preventive methods employed, and by creating awareness in the public through media. But tension headaches, migraine, dizziness, and malaise have become common presenting symptoms. It is also possible to get neurological symptoms because of depression or anxiety.

1. ***Patient reports with a feeling of discomfort in the head and not necessarily the pain, can be termed as HEADACHE.***

...believed that the stimuli causing headaches arise in the walls of the blood ... Vasodilatation of dural arteries, displacement or traction on sensitive basal ...essels or dural sinuses evoke pain. The cause of most headaches can be best ...ated by full and accurate history and by routine general examination of the ...nt.

History should bring out the probable cause — the factors that precipitate the attack ...r those factors that aggravate and ameliorate the attack. Total duration of the attack and whether there are any accompaniments such as vomiting and visual or sensory disturbances. Are there any symptoms between the attacks? Any head injury, sinusitis, surgical manipulations, and loss of weight etc.?

In order to select a correct remedy it is necessary to obtain a correct totality of the headache through its location, sensation, modalities and concomitants. If we scan through the repertory we can get all those modifying factors.

We shall study the most frequently indicated remedies for headaches:

Belladonna: has a vascular headache, throbbing and hammering, worse from motion and better letting the hair down. The fullness and pain is mostly felt in the forehead, which is worse from noise, light, lying down and jar, and mostly in the afternoon. It is better by sitting in semi-erect position and pressure. Staring brilliant eyes, with wide dilated pupils. The headache is worse on the right side.

Argentum metallicum: the headache and dyspepsia is induced by mental agitation, nursing the sick, and mental exertion such as students developing headaches during their examinations. There is dull paroxysmal neuralgia over the left side gradually increasing and suddenly ceasing. Head feels empty and hollow.

Bryonia alba: has bursting, splitting headache, worse by motion, stooping and opening the eyes, and when constipated. Headaches settle at occiput, and frontal ache is when frontal sinuses are involved. Scalp is very sensitive. Patient is irritable, and the aggravation is from motion and movement of any kind.

Gelsemium: sensation of band around the occiput, with a dull and heavy ache, heavy eyelids. Pain in the temples extending into the ears, associated with the muscular soreness of the shoulder and neck. They are preceded by blindness, better by profuse urination. Must want to keep his head raised over the pillow. In the congestive stage of meningitis there is pain in the back of the head with dilated pupils.

Glonoine: has cerebral congestion that causes throbbing and bursting headache. Headache that increases and decreases with the sun, giving waves of terrible pounding headache. Headache either before, during, after, or in place of menses. But the headache is better after sleep.

Kali bichromicum: has headaches in small spots, and often these headaches come on due to suppressed catarrh, over the eyebrows, preceded by blurred vision. The headache is worse from cold, that is better by pressing at the root of the nose and by drinking warm soup. The bones of the head feel sore with sharp stitches in bones, headache often associated with the sinusitis, that is having thick ropy sticky greenish yellow discharge.

Lachesis: has headache mostly at the time of menopause, heavy bursting down the nose, sensation as if the right side is cut off. The migraine pain extends to the neck and shoulder with pressure or burning of the vertex. Worse after moving. Sun aggravates this headache causing glimmering in vision, with flickering, dim vision, and pale face. Head is so sensitive that slight touch to the hair is unbearable. Modalities are very important, better by cold drinks, worse from alcohol, hot drinks, worse from sleep, after sleep, menopause, suppressed discharges, and better after appearance of discharges.

Natrum muriaticum: has migraine headaches, maddening, blinding, aches as if thousand little hammers were knocking on the brain, worse from awakening in the morning, at sunrise to sunset, during, before, or after menses, headache of school girls due to anaemia, slightest motion of eyes, while reading, frowning of fore-head can bring on headache. Frontal sinusitis can give this type of headache.

Pulsatilla: has headache from overwork. Suppressed sexual desire, indigestion, icecream. Better on walking in the open air. Pulsatilla is moody, with ever-changing symptoms, locations etc.

If you see the remedies detailed above for the headaches, you will note that all of them are polychrest remedies, that means one will have to consider their constitutional characters when selecting the remedy. Their usefulness will increase both in acute and chronic situations.

Repertory will provide one with more remedies mentioned under different locations, sensations and modalities.

2. ***An elderly person complains of severe paroxysms of knife-like or electric shock-like pain, lasting seconds, pain commencing in the mandibular division that spreads to the maxillary division of the fifth nerve and, at times to the ophthalmic division. These paroxysms are brought on by specific stimulation as trivial as washing, shaving, cold wind, or eating. This is neuralgia of fifth cranial nerve — TRIGEMINAL NEURALGIA.***

As usual, history taking is important. One has to determine whether the malady is of recent origin or a long standing, inherited or acquired. In elderly, as in the above case, degenerative changes must have already set in. But cases of neuralgia in persons who are still young will need antipsorics and acute remedies.

Aconite: is quite an invaluable remedy in very recent cases especially when caused by exposure to dry cold wind, the neuralgia is especially on the left side with restlessness, tingling and numbness. There is emotional and mental tension as shown in fright or fear and consequently anxiety and fear of death.

Belladonna: face becomes red and pale alternately, hot swollen and shiny, with twitching of muscles, Spasmodic distortion of face. Sensitive to light noise or to motion or to touch.

Colocynth: has long lasting action on trifacial nerves. The pains are accompanied by nausea, and patient vomits because of the intensity of the pain. These neuralgic pains are cutting, pinching, clamping, gnawing, followed by numbness, better by pressure. Specially suited to persons who are ill- humoured and who get easily angered.

Spigelia: Neuralgia of the fifth nerve is a common occurence. Very sensitive to touch. Worse from touch and stooping. The pain can suddenly disappear and reappear again.

Sanguinaria: will have periodic sick headache pains beginning in the occiput, spreads upwards or ascending over to the right eye. Fasting aggravates this headache. It is better by passing copious urine. And these headaches often return at menopause. The veins of the temple get distended; this headache also gets aggravated one to rising of the sun.

China: bursting and throbbing pain with throbbing of carotids. Sensation of bruised pain in the head. This headache is relieved with pressure and warm room but are worse in open air, in the sun, by contact, current of air, stepping. The scalp is sensitive to touch and combing.

Gelsemium: there is feeling of band around the occiput better by compression and keeping the head high. The pain in the temples extends into the ears, preceded by blindness; muscular soreness of the neck and shoulders. The headache is relieved by profuse urination.

Iris Versicular: headache that begins with the blurring of vision and by relaxing after strenuous work; with diarrhoea. It is better by gentle motion.

Melilotus: blood rushes to the head. The headache is violent, throbbing and congestive, and periodical. Headaches are better by nose bleed, or menstrual flow. The neuralgia is over the right side of the neck and head, and often alternates with backache; very trivial things often provoke the headache.

3. ***A young patient reports with involuntary movement of both the eyes and no other symptoms. The condition is NYSTAGMUS.***

Nystagmus is the rhythmic oscillation of the eyes. It is the sign of the disease of either the ocular or the vestibular system and its connections. It is described as either pendular or jerk. These movements must be sustained and demonstrable within binocular gaze.

The pendular movements are to and fro, similar both in the velocity and amplitude. It is always binocular, horizontal, and present in all directions of gaze. It is the disease of the vestibulo-cochlear nerve (Eighth Cranial nerve.)

Involuntary eye movements from side to side like a pendulum:

Agaricus: acompanying body symptoms are vertigo, marked and persistent with constant impulse to fall backward, twitching about eyes and face, redness without heat, puffy and distorted. Reading is difficult, as the types seem to swim, often a double vision, dim and flickering. Spasms of accommodation, twitching of eyelids, and eyeballs. Narrowing of space between the eyelids.

Carboneum hydrogenisatum: steady and extreme oscillation of the eyeball, eyes are distorted, lids are half closed, dark bodies move in front of the eyes. Pupils are insensible to light, vertigo is worse on going to open air.

Cuprum met: it affects the nerves of the cerebrospinal axis and muscles causing spasmodic effects — convulsions and cramps of violent form. Aching over the eyes, fixed staring, sunken glistening, turned upwards. The eyeballs rotate quickly behind the closed lids or roll from side to side. Bruised pain in the orbits, worse on moving the eyes.

Cicuta ver: patient persistently stare at the objects, strabismus, spasmodic movements after a fall or blow, letters go up and down or disappear when reading. Effects of exposure to snow. Eyes roll, jerk and stare. Eyelids twitch.

Zinc met: Ptosis and rolling of eyes. Blurring of one half of the vision, worse by stimulants. Squinting, Itching and soreness of lids and inner angles. Restless feet and continuous motion, cannot keep them still.

4. ***A young adult with a family history of recurrent paroxysms of unilateral spreading head pains, photophobia and biliousness preceded by transitory visual aura, the condition is probably MIGRAINE.***

Migraine or Sick Headache or Bilious Attack are paroxysmal and recurrent attacks of headaches. These attacks last from four to forty-eight hours or longer. In a typical migraine attack two phases are distinguished — the aura and the headache. The aura lasts for about 15/20 minutes. The commonest aura is the visual aura consisting of glittering zigzag lines curved or straight usually in one half of the field. The headaches succeed or is along with the aura but it never precedes. The headache starts in one of the frontal regions spreading to the opposite side of the head. But often it remains confined to one half of the head. It is accompanied by photophobia, flushing, pallor, vomiting or faint feelings. The pain lasts as said earlier for about 48 hours and leaves the person exhausted.

Treatment of Migraine will be considered in two phases — Acute Migraine attack and Chronic migraine attack. For treating the acute attack it will be necessary to have the acute totality of the attack which will comprise of (i) Cause or ailments from, (ii) sensations and any apparent pathology present, (iii) modalities including periodicity and other conditions of aggravation and amelioration, (iv) any strong concomitant.

After grief: Ignatia, Nat mur, Causticum

After Head Injury: Natrum sulph

Periodicity is another factor that is important modality.

Everyday: Arsenic alb, Belladonna

Day earlier each day: Formalin

Everyday same hour: Cedron and Kali Bich

Every seven days: China, Iris, Lac def. Sanguinaria, Silicea

Sul. Tuberculinum

Every eight days: Iris

Every fourteen days: Arsenic, Chelidonium, China

Sulphur and Tuberculinum

Every fourteen days and lasting for two or three days: Ferrum

Every six weeks: Magnesium mur.

In fact, history-taking is very important and any factor that attracts you as an important and peculiar modality should be thoroughly examined.

While treating chronic attacks of migraine, in addition to the above, one should get acquainted with the past history, the past attacks and various factors that have precipitated the same — constitutional characteristics and family idiosyncrasy. ***Natrum Muriaticum*** shows a very close resemblance to the malady, the other remedies should be studied in order to prepare the chronic picture of the case.

While studying the Chronic picture close to the chronic malady are ***Argentum nitricum, Arsenic alb, Chamomilla , Causticum*** **and *China.***

While treating these cases attention should be paid to the psychological and environmental factors, otherwise the treatment may not be of good use. Very often the cause of these attacks lie in teeth, sinuses, or in uncorrected errors of refraction. In older patients, cervical spondylitis may be one of the causes.

5. ***A patient complains of vertigo, faint feeling, apathy or depression and shows sweating, pallor, flushing of face, and tachycardia, vomiting occurring only at sea, in cars, trains, elevators, round-abouts, swings, or flying. The condition is MOTION SICKNESS.***

The cause of this feeling is the effect of acceleration, linear, angular, vertical etc., on the labyrinths. This is common in subjects of frequent migraine attacks. These may persist for some time after the cause but may settle down. The adults adapt to air travel. Rest in bed is advised and very light food is given in little quantity.

Cocculus indicus: is the most useful remedy. Sick headache from carriage riding, with sense of emptiness in the head. Pain in the occiput is worse on lying on the head, and is better bending backwards. Aversion to food, but there is desire for cold drinks. Along with vertigo there is nausea and vomiting which is closely related to car or sea sickness. Palpitation worse in the morning. It also helps the sensitive condition caused by loss of sleep, night watching.

Petroleum: the vertigo and heaviness are often associated with nausea and bilious vomiting. This nausea with or without vomiting is one of the grand characteristics of this remedy and it is worse by motion in a carriage, car, or at sea. It is one of the first remedies to be thought of in train sickness or sea sickness.

Conium maculatum: is an old person's remedy, worse from seeing moving objects and alcohol. Turning in bed causes vertigo. Vertigo on lying down and turning over in bed. Turning head sideways or turning eyes, worse on shaking head.

6. ***The patient complains of recurrent vertigo, associated with deafness, and tinnitus. It is either MENIERE'S SYNDROME or OTOSCLEROSIS.***

It occurs between the age of 30 and 60. The attacks of acute labyrinthine failure are paroxysmal with recurrent vertigo and vomiting and each attack leaves the patient with increasing deafness, and between the attacks there is tinnitus in the affected ear. The disease is bilateral but one side may get affected first. In Otosclerosis there is gradually increasing deafness commencing at an early age. 'Paracusis' — an ability to hear in noisy surrounding — is more marked. Tinnitus is marked but giddiness is uncommon.

China sulph: acts on the nerves causing great sensitiveness to external influences. There is a periodical neuralgia, and tinnitus. Violent ringing, buzzing and roaring in the ears, with occasional deafness of the same side. Often this is associated with violent headache. The preparation of China salicylicum is the most injurious to the structure of internal ear and there Cozzolino, in all likelihood, is a very powerful homoeopathic cure.

In **Phosphorus:** there is difficulty in hearing human voice. There are echoes and reverberations of sounds, especially music. There is a constant feeling that there is obstruction in front of ears, as if a foreign body

Theridion: has a peculiar symptom , has an extreme hypersensitiveness of nerves and, therefore, very hypersensitive to noise, which penetrates the body.

Silicea: there is perforated drum, deafness and also hears with a loud report, worse in full moon, roaring in the ears, hissing noises, feeling of stoppage in ear, better when swallowing or yawning.

Salicylic acid: has auditory nerve vertigo, with troublesome nausea accompanying head symptoms. Hearing is diminished. Deafness, with noises in the ear. Roaring and ringing in the ears, deafness with vertigo. Buzzing of flies or bees.

7. ***Person is attacked with deep, persistent and prolonged unconsciousness, from which he cannot be roused by shaking or calling. The case is of COMA. (A lesser degree of coma is stupor).***

The coma is of sudden onset when there is head injury. Or due to haemorrhagic or embolic lesions within the brain substance.

It can also happen due to hypertensive attack, an occlusion of the cerebral vessel by thrombosis. It can also happen when a meningeal vessel bleeds or is in a hypoglycaemic condition.

If this coma persists after the night rest and sleep, the cause could be cerebral infarction or intoxication from hypnotics.

Assess the cause of the coma condition first by obtaining correct history from relatives, neighbours etc. Any preceding ill-health like Hypetrension, Diabetes mellitus, or, was the patient depressed or suicidal, (poisoning) or subject to headaches(cerebral neoplasm) Did this attack come suddenly (Cerebral haemorrhage)or gradually (hypoglycaemia). Usually Coma in childhood is due to Meningitis, Epilepsy or intracranial neoplasm or abscesses. In the middle age, suspect Cerebral haemorrhage.

Helleborus niger: develops coma and unconsciousness after a blow on the head resulting into concussion and when Arnica fails to relieve the situation. Rolls head from side to side with moaning if there is hydrocephalus. Bores the head into pillow for relief if he has meningeal fever; forehead wrinkled in folds in brain disorders: cold sweat. This comatose state can come on due to checked exanthemata, blows or disappointed love.

Hyoscyamus niger: There is erotic mania, inclined to laugh at everything. Muttering delirium. Low speech with constant carphologia with deep stupor. Can barely be aroused. Twitching of facial muscles is a grand characteristics, with unconsciousness.

Moschus: has violent anger, talks excitedly, raves, scolds. Coldness of the body or single parts is a characteristic until mouth becomes dry, lips blue, eyes staring and then falls unconscious.

The line of treatment will depend on the exact mode of its cause. Coma can be either due to head injury, or due to embolic or haemorrhagic lesion within the brain substance. First two remedies those come to our mind are Arnica and Natrum sulph and/or Opium.

Arnica: cures hemorrhages of any kind. Strokes, dilatation of blood vessels or rupture of small vessels. In short, hemorrhage into tissues of internal organs or the skin. Coldness of the nose is an odd symptom of Arnica. Trauma and its effects, recent or remote, including mental shock. Characteristic is when spoken to answers correctly but relapses; there is muttering delirium.

Natrum sulph: has ill-effects of falls and injuries to the head, or the mental or physical troubles start later. Whenever he returns to senses complains of sensations as if the forehead would burst, as if a screw is being driven in, as if the brain is loose in side as bells are ringing in the ears.

Opium: all complaints are characterized by stupor, although the complaints are painless. And are accompanied by heavy deep sleep, stertorous breathing, sweaty skin. Face turns dark mahogany brown venous passive congestion and effects of stroke. Pupils contract. Ill-effects of fear, fright, anger, shame, sudden joy, sun and drug overdose. Worse from stimulants.

Belladonna: is extremely hypersensitive to light, touch and noise; has widely dilated pupils, staring and brilliant eyes, complains of throbbing headache.

Gelsemium: centers in its action on the muscles and nerves In muscles it causes overpowering aching, tiredness, heaviness, weakness, and soreness. Dizziness, dullness and trembling. There is complete relaxation and dullness, prostration. Bad effects from fright, fear, exciting news, dread of falling, fear of doctors and dentists. Closes his eyes but is very conscious. Although he finds very difficult to keep his eyes open.

Zincum: the word fatigue covers a large part of its action. Zinc is too weak to develop exanthema, or menstrual function, to expectorate, to urinate, or to understand to remember. There is restlessness in the limbs, and and cannot keep them still.

8. ***Person experiences a sudden disturbance of consciousness with convulsion and falling. It is an EPILEPTIC SEIZURE.***

Epilepsy by definition is the continuing tendency to have such seizures, even if a long interval separates these attacks.

There are many anticonvulsive remedies of repute, but we will consider only those which are commonly indicated in clinical practice. The rest of them can be studied from the repertorial presentations.

Our available remedies are from vegetable kingdom : The three umbelliferae: Oenantha crocata, Cicuta verosa, and Aethusa cynapium; and Belladonna of Solanaceae and Absinthinum from compositae. From chemical kingdom we can mention Copper, Plumbum, and Arsenic. Although these following drugs have not produced typical epileptiform seizures, they have shown their overexcitablity of the nervous centers. Strychnine, Nux vom, Ignatia, Calcarea and Silicea. Hydrocyanic acid has proved to have a close resemblance to the epileptic seizure.

Oenantha crocata: has epileptic convulsions and worse during convulsions, and pregnancy. Convulsive twitching of the facial muscles, foaming at the mouth, falls backwards and utters a loud cry before falling. Coma follows the convulsion. Averse to be questioned.

Cicuta verosa: has chief influence on the brain, medulla oblongata, nervous system and gastrointestinal tract, and the skin. Action induces spasmodic affections. C. verosa, corresponds to falls and effects of concussion-like convergent strabismus, sudden rigidity, then jerks and violent distortions followed by prostration. Jerking of left arm all day. We find this in the very nervous, in children and elderly persons. Head is turned and twisted to one side.

Aethusa cynapium: affects the brain and nervous system which is connected with the gastro-intestinal system. Anguish, cry, expression of uneasiness, and discontent, mostly during teething process in children and during summer. The thumbs are clenched, face becomes red, eyes turned downwards, pupils dilated, and staring; there is often foam at the mouth. Inability to digest milk.

Absinthinum: the convulsions are preceded by trembling, makes grimaces, bites tongue and foam at the mouth. At times there is severe sudden giddiness, delirium with delusions and loss of consciouness and after an attack there is transient loss of memory. Often used in tincture and followed by 3c.

Cuprum met.: it affects the nerves of the cerebrospinal axis and muscles, causing spasmodic effect, convulsions, and cramps of violent form. It has a great nausea; greater than any other remedy. Cramps begin in the fingers and toes, violent contractive and intermitting pain. Chorea from fright. Aura begins in the knee, ascends to hypogastrium, then unconsciousness, foaming and falling. Convulsions are either tonic or clonic. In children during dentition, children lie on abdomen and jerk the buttocks up. Cramps in toes, fingers and calves.

Artemisia vulgaris: Patient is excitable and irritable before an attack. The attack of epilepsy is brought on after a fright or grief, after a blow on the head, with menstrual disturbances during teething. The attack is accompanied by profuse offensive sweat or seminal ejaculation. The sweat has a peculiar garlic odour. The attacks are usually repeated after long intervals of rest. Worms can also bring on these attacks. Excessive masturbatory activity also brings on these attacks. In the attack the mouth is drawn towards the left, chewing movements, grinding teeth, difficult to utter words.

9. *A child with fever, develops sudden convulsions — a state of FEBRILE CONVULSIONS.*

Febrile convulsions in infancy has less serious significance than in adult life. The convulsion threshold appears to be lower in infancy and that increases with the maturation of the nervous system. In infancy the febrile states such as teething, exanthemata, gastro-intestinal infections are frequent and common causes of convulsions. A single fit occurs, there is little cause for alarm but if there is repeated attacks in recurrent illness or if they appear without any adequate cause, then Epilepsy is the likely diagnosis.

Examine the child thoroughly and determine the cause of convulsion. The treatment shall be to control the convulsion and reduce the fever. Immerse the child in warm water bath for about 10 minutes, then place the child in a warm bed. Look for rash on the body, any source of sepsis (throat and ears) examine the chest. Look for any head retraction, squint or Kernig's sign and lastly examine the stools and urine.

Belladonna: there is sudden high fever with hot head, cold limbs and delirium. Perspiration is only on the head and there is no thirst with the fever. Pupils are dilated, eyes are staring, brilliant conjunctiva with a staring look. Jerks and spasm in the limbs. Perspiration on the head and there is no thirst with the fever. The skin is moist and dry alternately.

Artemisia vulgaris: is indicated in convulsions of nervous mothers or teething children. Cooling off while getting heated from dancing or exertion, from menstrual disturbances, and goes into deep sleep after the attack.

Bufo rana: has convulsive seizures, they occur mostly at night in sleep, This is often associated with disturbance of sexual sphere, seizures occur during menstrual flow, when the sexual desire is excited in young men, or during sex. These attacks are followed by headaches. Convulsions can come in children after nursing frightened mother or angry mother.

Causticum: has convulsions due to suppressed eruptions, Ailments from long-lasting grief and develops mental fatigue. Laughs before or after the spasm.

Cicuta verosa: Convulsions occur due to concussions, with sudden shocks through head; neck muscles get contracted. Foam in and around the mouth, grinding of teeth with lock-jaw. Twitching and spasmodic jerks, are the keynote of cicuta. The patient is better by dark and quiet room.

Zinc metallicum: has trembling convulsive twitching and fidgety feet; worse at night, during sleep and from spinal injuries; there are automatic movements of mouth, arms and hands.

10. ***A person complains of intense malaise, fever, rigors, severe headache, photophobia and vomiting. He is irritable and prefers to lie still and has neck stiffness and subsequently develops a positive Kernig's sign. He is suffering from MENINGITIC SYNDROME.***

In meningitis, the infection can be caused by bacteria, viruses, or fungi. In meningococcal infection there will be petechial rash; in Pneumococcal infection there is often a skull fracture, ear disease, or a congenital CNS lesion. Leptospirosis is responsible in cases who are working in drains, canals polluted rivers etc.

Acute bacterial meningitis is recognized by its sudden onset, rigors and high fever. A petechial rash may be present which is a strong evidence of the disease. Viral meningitis is benign self-limiting, lasting for about 4-10 days. Headache may follow but there are no sequelae. Tubercular meningitis causes a chronic meningitis commencing with vague headache, lassitude, anorexia and vomiting. Meningitic signs may appear after few days or weeks.

Meningitis is an emergency, and when untreated is lettial. CT scan and Lumbar puncture should be carried out to study CSF (Cerebro Spinal Fluid).

Apis mellifica: is the first rank remedy in this condition. The pathogenesis of Apis mostly corresponds to the meningeal condition. The patient is nervous, restless and oversensitive or hot or drowsy with or without thirst, Worse from pressure or touch to head, very sensitive to heat or heated warm rooms. and better by cold water, thirst during chill, burning heat but feels chilly when moved. Stupor with sudden short cries. There is great fidgetiness. Stiffness being accompanied by feeling of constriction.

Helliborus niger: Hahnemann's observation is that it has kind of stupor dullness of sensorium, a condition that there is nothing wrong with eyes but that he cannot see anything and patient does ot pay attention to anything. There is a sensorial depression and at times complete unconsciousness, involuntary sighing. Picks up clothes and at lips. Rolling of the head constantly. Bores the head into the pillow for relief than headache. There is neck rigidity, stiffness and painful sensibility, swelling of the glands of the neck.

Gelsemium: has a very characteristic headache, beginning in the occiput and spreading over the whole head, sailing over the eyes. Dizziness and dim vision rising from the occiput over the head, depression from the heat of summer. Headache is with stiffness of the neck which is worse in the morning and is better by urinating. Headache is preceded by blurring before the eyes, drowsiness with headache, difficulty in keeping the eyes open. There is chill running up and down the back, and similar condition present in Influenza, cerebrospinal fever.

Stramonium: develops headache with incoherent talk. Raises head frequently from the pillow and drops it again in unconscious and delirious state. Pain in forehead and over the eyebrows beginning at 9 am in the morning which is worse till the afternoon.This is common in meningitis from suppressed ear discharge.

11. ***Usually a middle-aged person between the age of 20-40 years suddenly gets pain in the back which occurs after strenuous activity, typically with back in the forward flexion. The pain is aggravated by movement and by certain activity. The condition is Intervertebral DISC DISEASE or SCIATICA.***

This term disc disease describes an acute syndrome where there is a disc prolapse causing a condition which is usually known as lumbago or sciatica, depending on the presence of involvement of sciatic nerve. It is also known as the chronic degenerative change, and then the condition is called spondylosis. Most commonly the three lowest dics are involved — L5/S1, L4/L5, and L4/L3 discs. In mild cases there is no sign but the characteristic findings include compensatory scoliosis, and limitation of movements in all direction.

More than medicinal treatment is required rest for few days on a firm bed. Lumbar belt or corset should be used in the recovery stage. Physiotherapy to relieve pain should be suggested. However, certain homoeopathic remedies can be of some use.

Colocynth: has a long lasting action on the large nerves especially Trifacial, sciatica, and spinal. There is heavy weight in lumbar and dorsal regions which is better on lying on the left side. The pain may extend into the right scapula, better by pressure. Cramp-like pain in the hip, better lying on the affected side. The neck becomes stiff which is worse on moving the head. In the hip there is cramp-like pain, with contraction of the muscles. The sciatic pain is worse on the left side better by pressure heat.

Gnaphalium: There is an intense pain along the sciatic nerve and this pain alternates with numbness, worse on lying down, motion and stepping, better by flexing the legs on abdomen. Or by sitting in the chair. Frequent pains in the calves and feet. Feeling of weakness, incapable of lifting the slightest weight.

Kali Iodatum: the pains are worse on lying on the affected side, pain is more marked in the small of the back and coccyx. Pain in the hips forcing limping, better by walking and flexing legs, formication of the lower limbs when sitting, better by lying down. The sciatica is worse at night, and worse lying on the painful side.

Nux vomica: pain in the back causes him to drag the feet. Unsteady gait, with feeling of stiffness, with the sensation of sudden loss of power in the legs, with cramps in the calves and soles.

Tellurium metallicum: there is weak feeling in the back. Pain in the last cervical to fifth dorsal vertebra. Sensitive spinal column to touch, straining, and at night. Lumbar pain in the right thigh, better by walking.

Rhus toxicodendron: stiffneck with painful tension, when moving, pain and stiffness in the small of the back, better by motion and on lying on hard support, worse while sitting. Coccyx aches into the thighs.

12. ***There is more or less sudden paralysis affecting one side of the body, motor sensory, visual or speech functions are affected. The condition is STROKE***

It is a cerebral vascular attack usually due to disease of the intracranial vessels, although the cause is extracranial, such as embolism, carotid or vertebral occlusion, essential or renal hypertension, haemorrhagic diseases or pyemia. Hemiplegia is the commonest manifestation of stroke.

Arnica: is disposed to cerebral congestion. Strokes with red face, and great prostration with tired feeling in sanguine plethoric persons. Hot head with cold body, confusion and sensitiveness in brain with sharp pinching pains. Arnica is suited to all kinds of strokes, dilatation and rupture of small blood vessels causing extravasation of blood in the tissues. An odd sensation is coldness of the nose.

Glonoin: here the cerebral congestion is due to elevated blood pressure, which often sends the patient in convulsion. The face is bright red and puffed, the pulse is full and hard, and the urine is albuminous. There is often sudden fainting, with black spots in front of the eyes and sudden onset of unconsciousness. Both Glonoin and Belladonna have congestion and inflammation of the brain. Head symptoms are worse by bending the head backwards, worse in winter, and from application of cold water. Belladonna has relief from bending backward and sitting up with head quiet.

Hyoscyamus: the symptoms point to weakness and nervous agitation, with coma vigil. Tremulous weakness and twitching of tendons. Spasmodic affections generally with delirium. Makes gestures, carphology, picks bed clothes with fingers. Convulsions, trembling, jerking, twitching and cramps are marked features. There is active mania with alternation that ends in deep sopor. Also useful in eclampsia, chorea, local twitching of solitary muscle. Muttering delirium. There is involuntary urination because of bladder paralysis.

Belladonna: has vascular headache, throbbing, hammering headache, worse in the temples and worse by movements, better by bending head backwards. Pain worse by noise, light, better by pressure. It acts on the nerve center producing twitching, convulsions and pain. It produces active congestion, furious excitement, congestion that follows vascular exacerbation in the brain due to haemorrhage.

Hemiplegia is the commonest manifestation of a "stroke" with paralysis affecting the face. If the responsible cerebral lesion is acute the paralysis at first is flaccid. But in complete hemiplegia the arm is affected more than the legs and the distal movements are affected more than the proximal ones. In the phase of recovery — residual hemiplegia — spasticity of the affected limb is of clasp knife variety.

Most cases of acute hemiplegia is due to cerebro-vascular accidents. Causticum, Rhustox, Lachesis, and Phosphoric acid are mostly indicated. The description of these remedies in paralysis may be rad elsewhere in the book.

13. **Patient complains of pain behind the ears, and in front of the mastoid, lymphatic gland is palpable behind the angle of the jaw and the onset of paralysis is very rapid. Stiffness of the affected side, and cannot close the eyes properly and tears flow from the flaccid lower lid. The condition is *BELL'S PALSY*.**

Causticum: is primary remedy to think of in such case. The facial paralysis is caused because of the cold drought, neuralgia of the right cheek bones, to mastoid process, worse at night. Jaw joints are affected with rheumatism. Sickly, shallow, low-spirited expression. Patient is better in damp cold weather but aggravated in fine but cold weather. Causticum has paralysis of the single parts.

Agaricus: there is facial twitching, muscles feel stiff, face itches and burns. Lancinating and tearing pains in the cheek as of splinters. Neuralgia as if of cold needles, running through nerves or sharp ice touched them. Grimaces, idiotic expression, face is blue and puffed.

Belladonna: face becomes pale and red alternately, hot, swollen, and shining, swelling of the upper lip, facial neuralgia with twitching muscles and flushed face. There is spasmodic distortion of the mouth. Convulsive motions of the muscles of the face, lower jaw is as drawn backwards.

Gelsemium: centers its action upon muscles and motor nerves. In muscles, it causes overpowering, aching, tiredness, heaviness, weakness and soreness. It causes various degrees of motor paralysis, cold and dampness brings on many complaints. In the face hot, heavy, flushed, besotted-looking expression. Facial muscles are contracted, especially around the mouth. Lower jaw wags sideways.

14. ***Patient complains of bilateral or unilateral root pains and paraesthesiae extending from neck, down the arms, to the fingers involving more than one cervical root, sometimes wasting, of the intrinsic muscles of the hands and reduced tendon reflexes. There is often a chronic neck stiffness, with characteristic degenerative changes in X-rays of the cervical spine. The condition is probably CERVICAL SPONDYLOSIS.***

This is also known as cervical osteoarthritis. Onset mostly after the age of fifty but earlier not ruled out. This is due to degenerative condition affecting the middle and lower cervical vertebrae. There is painful stiffness of the neck with painful creaking and grating on movements. The area of pain differs on the basis of the nerve roots that are affected. There are periods of remissions and recurrences are common. Medicinal treatment is not of much value, it may reduce the pain but not fully cure. The only useful treatment for these patients is exercise under supervision of a qualified physiotherapist and short wave diathermy. Pain-killers may not help but may reduce the suffering.

Paris quadrifolia: develops a weight and weariness in the nape of the neck and across shoulders. Neuralgia begins in the left intercostal region extending into the left arm. Joints feel broken swollen or dislocated at every motion. Numbness of the upper limb and fingers.

Ranunculus bulbosus: chest is the seat of these pains. Muscular pains on the origins of the scapula, in women of sedentary habits. Pains are often burning in spots. Particularly from needlework, type-writing and piano playing. The pains are more marked while writing, in writer's cramp and professional neurosis. Patient is better by standing, sitting bent forwards, worse from open air, damp cold rainy and stormy weather, change of position and motion of arms.

Rhus Toxicodendron: it affects the fibrous tissue, markedly joints. Tendon sheaths producing pains and stiffness. Usually after overstraining, lifting, and wet weather while perspiring. The pains are shooting, tearing and stitching, worse at night and cannot rest in any position.

15. ***Middle-aged woman complains of fatiguability, particularly in the proximal limb muscles and the muscles of mastication. It is mostly a case of MYESTHENIA GRAVIS.***

This is an acquired condition characterized by weakness and fatiguability of the proximal limb, ocular and bulbar muscles. The heart is not affected. Complex extra-ocular palsies, ptosis and typical fluctuating proximal weakness are found. The cause is unknown. The IgG antibodies to acetylcholine receptors are found. The prognosis is not favourable.

Alumina: this is a remedy for elderly and feeble patients, especially in senile dementia. There is great general fatigue even after a short walk but chiefly after speaking. Frequent stretching while sitting and drags the leg, especially the left one. Sluggishness of action is the characteristic of this remedy. Staggers on walking, the legs feel numb. Heels feel numb when stepping. Spinal degeneration and paralysis of the lower limbs.

Conium: has difficult gait, trembling and sudden loss of strength while walking with painful stiffness of the legs etc. It affects the nerves and muscles causing incoordination, and paralysis, uncertain gait and difficult speech. Great progressive debility in the morning in bed, and has a general feeling of bruised as if beaten. Paralysis of ocular muscles, heavy droop, worse outside, excessive lachrymation without inflammation. Myopia is not uncommon. Muscular weakness, especially of the lower limbs, walks very comfortably with eyes closed but staggers, becomes giddy and nauseated when walking with open eyes. Shortness of breath on least exertion.

Gelsemium: it centers its action on the muscles and the motor nerves. In the muscles it causes overpowering aching, tiredness, heaviness, weakness and soreness. Fatigue after slight exercise, professional neurosis, writer's cramp, heavy lower limbs, knees weak and worse descending, tottering gait. Muscles of the mouth seem contracted.

16. ***An young adult complains of sudden drag in the feet, and the arm has become suddenly useless, and that there is a double vision. The condition is probably MULTIPLE SCLEROSIS (or disseminated sclerosis).***

It is due to scattered areas of demyelination in the spinal cord, brain stem, optic nerve and cerebellum appearing at intervals, over many years, commencing between the age of 20-45 years.

The presenting symptom is sudden loss of power in arm or leg but other initial complaints are also common, like double vision, or sudden unilateral blindness, numbness and tingling etc. Their essential characters are that the lesions develop acute symptoms at irregular interval and have scattered distribution.

There is no curative treatment of this potentially disabling disease. Once diagnosed the patient should be informed about the disease. And long term planning for employment, home and plans for the future should be considered.

Causticum: acts upon the nerves, motor and sensory, and on the voluntary and involuntary muscles of bladder, larynx and limbs. There is increasing loss of muscular strength, causing uncertainty of the control over the muscles and finally ending in the paralysis of a single organ or the parts. Manifests its action mainly in chronic rheumatism, arthritic and paralytic disorders. Burning, rawness and soreness are the characteristics. Paralysis of ocular muscles after exposure to cold, paralysis of one eyelid, weakness of recti muscles, diplopia, better looking at the right, vision obscured as if from gauze, sparks and dark spots before the eyes. Twisting and jerking in limbs. Burning in joints, unsteady walking and easily falling, weak ankles, and restless legs at night.

Gelsemium: It centers is action on the motor nerves and the muscles. In muscles it causes overpowering aching, tiredness, weakness and soreness — mostly in the limbs. There is complete relaxation and prostration. It acts on the nervous system, causes various degrees of motor paralysis, cold and dampness brings on many complaints. Lack of muscular coordination, and children have the fear of falling and they grab the crib or the nurse. Heavy drooping eyelids, Ptosis and hardly opens the eyes. Blurring and discomfort in eyes even after accurately adjusted glasses. Vision is blurred and smoky. There is loss of power in the limbs, and lack of muscle control, excessive trembling and weakness of all the limbs. Descending tottering gait and cannot direct his legs.

Burning, rawness and soreness are the characteristics. Paralysis of ocular muscles after exposure to cold paralysis of one eyelid, weakness of recti muscles, diplopia, better looking at the right, vision obscured as if from gauze, sparks and dark spots before the eyes. Twisting and jerking in limbs. Burning in joints, unsteady walking and easily falling, weak ankles, and restless legs at night.

Lathyrus sativus: It affects the anterior and lateral columns of the cord, producing many paralytic conditions. Excessive rigidity of legs. And develops spastic gait. Heels do not touch the ground while walking. Muscles of the lower extremity and the gluteal muscles are emaciated. Cannot extend or cross legs when sitting. The legs are cold during the day and burning hot during night.

17. ***A patient reports with pyrexia, followed by flaccid paralysis of one or more limbs. He does not have any sensory changes. The condition may be ACUTE POLIOMYELITIS.***

Although no age is exempt major incidence is in children between two and ten years. It is a viral infection having an incubation period of three days to five weeks. This virus has a selective affinity for the ventral horn cells of spinal cord, their motor homologues in the bulb and the reticular substance of the pons. This results in loss of power and flaccid paralysis, more or less widespread, recovery may occur in partially damaged cells.

In about 40% of cases there is minor illness with fever and sore throat, headache or nasal catarrh. The disease can be aborted at this stage. In other cases this may be followed by major illness — pre-paralytic or paralytic stages. The pre-paralytic stage closely resembles Influenza. With severe headache, backache, pains in the chest, abdomen and thighs, sore throat, vomiting or diarrhoea and there may be joint pains. It is quite remarkable that the consciouness is fully preserved whist the neurological symptoms are developing.

This comes in epidemic form and hospitalization is advised to avoid any serious complication. The patient needs absolute physiological, emotional and physical rest.

Aconite, Arnica, Rhustox, and Gelsemium are often indicated in the early phase of pre-paralytic stage. Introduction of these remedies at appropriate time often help to abort the disease.

Gelsemium: has a action on the muscles and the motor nerves and causes overpowering muscle ache, tiredness, heaviness, weakness and soreness especially felt in the limbs. The typical drowsiness, heavy stupid sleep, and yawning are common.

There is loss of power of muscular control, trembling, weakness of all the limbs. Feeling of partial luxation of patella, when walking and fatigue after slight exertion. Fever with a stupor, dizziness, faintness, thirstless and prostrated. During 1955-56, in epidemic of Influenza which spread countrywide, Gelsemium and Eupatorium were the mainstay in the absence of any remedy with modern medicine.

Lathyrus: affects the anterior and the lateral columns of the cord causing many paralytic disorders of the lower limbs. Gluteal muscles and the muscles of the lower extremities are emaciated. There is stiffness and lameness of the ankles and knees. Feet are dragged and or put down forcibly while walking. While lying down the limbs can be moved from side to side but cannot be lifted. The condition is worse in cold damp weather.

Plumbum met.: it is a great remedy for sclerotic condition affecting the muscles, nerves, spinal cord, abdomen. Plumbum has progressive muscular atrophy with excessive and rapid emaciation. The paralysis of single parts, wrist drop, flaccid with hyperesthesia, worse from touch. There is pain in the atrophied limbs, alternating with colic. Arms shake when attempting to use them.

A very optimistic programme of prevention of Polio has been taken up by WHO, there is strong belief that world can get rid off this infection in a very near future. Already the incidence of polio worldwide has come down drastically except in economically and socially poor countries.

12 CARDIOVASCULAR SYSTEM

- Cardinal Features of diseases of heart
- Percarditis
- Endocarditis
- Angina Pectoris
- Myocardial Infarction
- Acute rheumatic fever
- Hypertension
- Valvular diseases
- Dilatation of the heart
- Hypertrophy of the heart
- Intermittent claudication
- Superficial Thrombophlebitis

Cardinal Features of diseases of heart

Dyspnoea: It is increased awareness of breathlessness. It can be because of cardiac or respiratory causes. It can be a symptom also in healthy persons during exercise. It is clinically valuable to grade dyspnoea by the amount of physical exertion possible before breathlessness occurs, e.g. climbing 14 stairs or walking 200 yards flat.

Orthopnoea: It is form of breathlessness or dyspnoea that is experienced by the patient on lying down. This happens because lying flat results in redistribution of blood leading to an increased central and pulmonary blood volume.

Chest pain: It is gripping or crushing central chest pain or discomfort that may be felt around the whole chest or deep within the chest.

Palpitation: It is the increased awareness of the normal heart beat, or the sensation of the slow or rapid heart rate or an irregular heart rhythm. **Syncope:** It is due to many causes. But the cardiovascular syncope is usually sudden and brief. Without warning, the patient falls to ground, looks pale and becomes deeply unconscious. The pulse is usually slow and at times absent. In a few seconds the position flashes back and recovers from the unconsciousness and the pulse quickens. Cardiac arrhythmia or valvular or vascular obstruction.

Fatigue: This tiredness and lethargy is associated with heart failure, persistent cardiac arrhythmia, or cyanotic heart disease .It is due to poor oxygenation or cerebral or peripheral perfusion.

Oedema: Heart failure results in salt and water retention and this retained fluid accumulates in the limbs in the ambulant patient and in the sacrum in the bed-bound patients.

1. ***There is a raised temperature, patient is in an evident distress, pericardial friction sound rub is audible. The condition is ACUTE PERICARDITIS.***

On examination we find precordial area of dullness is increased, the shape of dullness being pyramidal with the point upwards. This condition is found associated with many acute diseases and specially rheumatic fever. This fever can come insidiously without pain or dullness. The typical constitutional symptoms like anxiety, distressing look, puffiness of the face, but not amounting to oedema. Rapid pulse and fever, rapid breathing, and pain in the left chest is noticed.

The commonest remedies to our mind at this point are Aconite, Arsenic alb, Apis.

Aconite: has a great fear, anxiety, distress is seen on the face, even fears of death. This ailment may even start with fear. The heart pains radiate to the left shoulder with tachycardia, and palpitation. The pulse is fast, full, hard and bounding.

Arsenic alb: restlessness and anguish is the character. Pains are in the heart and extend up to neck and occiput, with anxiety. The pulse is more rapid in the morning, and palpitation is worse lying on the back, and ascending steps. Visible pulsation and beats are audible. Mostly, these are smokers or tobacco-chewers.

Apis: is fussy and fidgety, Chest feels beaten and bruised. The heart beats shake the whole body, Stitching pains travel backwards from apex. Palpitation of the heart, scanty secretions of urine, the pulse is hard, small, intermittent and quick but weak. Often associated with organic heart disease. But during the second stage that follows this, within a day or two, there is effusion while pain and tenderness diminishes. Breathlessness and other symptoms continue, cough becomes more troublesome. The breathing becomes panting, short dry cough with supra-sternal pain. Apis still remains an indicated remedy.

Colchicum: complaints of old people. Asthmatics and of gouty constitution and uric acid diathesis. There is anxiety in the region of heart, pressure and oppression in the region of heart, sound in the heart becomes weaker and pulse of low tension, cutting and stinging of heart. The pulse is thready and imperceptible.

Kali carb: the mind is full of fear and imagination, particularly when alone. Very anxious about his disease condition. Violent palpitation shakes the whole body, throbbing, extending to the tip of the fingers. Heart pains radiate to the left shoulder, associated with arrhythmia.

Spigelia: specially adapted to anaemic, debilitated and rheumatic constitution. Violent palpitation, audible, and accompany symptoms of other diseases as well. Violent sticking, and or compressive pains, radiating to arms, throat and scapula. Craves for hot water that relieves. Rheumatic carditis, trembling pulse and the whole left side is sore. Precordial pains are aggravated by movements.

Duration and course of this pericarditis widely varies, but the average is about two to three weeks. It may undergo resolution with or without the formation of adhesions.

2. ***The patient is elderly, pale, often anaemic, and ill. Intermittently pyrexial and complains of myalgia, and arthralgia. The persistence of fever and development of heart murmurs after an acute suppurative illness like pneumonia or meningitis. ACUTE ENDOCARDITIS is suspected.***

Clinically, this endocarditis could be subacute endocarditis, but for the purpose of treatment remedies remain same. The remedies are listed under acute pericarditis. We consider some more remedies with the sphere of action on the cardiac pathology:

Aurum met. and Aurum mur. : These remedies should be considered usually when there is arteriosclerosis, high blood pressure, and nightly paroxysms of pain behind the sternum. Presence of valvular lesions of arteriosclerosis, with a sensation of heart being stopped beating for two or three seconds, followed by sinking sensation behind the epigastrium. Violent palpitation and oppression of the heart. The pulse is rapid, feeble and irregular, with visible throbbing of the carotid.

Kalmia latifolia: it is heart, nerve and rheumatic remedy. The heart's action is tumultuous, rapid and visible. There is anguish around the heart, fluttering of the heart, with anxiety. Pains are sharp and burning, shooting, radiating to left scapula, and the palpitation is worse on leaning forward. Often there will be gouty and rheumatic metastasis of heart. There is tachycardia with pain. The salient features are wandering rheumatic pain which travels from above downwards, tumultuous action of the heart and slow pulse.

Spigelia: has violent palpitations, audible, attending with symptoms of other diseases. Throbbing of carotids. Violent and sticking compressive type of pains. Soreness and purring of the heart. Pulse is trembling and rheumatic carditis. The whole left side is sore.

Veratrum viridae: constant dull burning pain in the region of the heart; there is beating of pulses throughout the body but the pulse is slow, soft and weak. Irregular and intermittent. Veratrum v., is known to produce violent congestive conditions. Induces fall in systolic and diastolic blood pressure. Paroxysms of auricular fibrillation.

After the treatment of Endocarditis a constitutional remedy should be prescribed to develop immunity.

3. ***A post-mid-life patient is attacked by constrictive pain in the chest The condition is ANGINA PECTORIS.***

Chest pain is the most classical symptom associated with ischaemia of the heart disease. Classical or exertional angina, that is related to exertion, especially after a meal, or in cold weather, or walking against the wind that provokes the pain. Also aggravated by anger or excitement. The pain vanishes promptly when the exertion stops.

Decubitus angina: that occurs when the patient lies down or takes a recumbent posture. This occurs in association with heart failure.

Nocturnal angina: This wakes the patient from sleep. May be provoked by vivid dreams. Patients with symptoms of critical coronary artery disease have this form.

Variant angina: (Prinzmetal's Angina): has no obvious provocation It occurs at rest, especially at night, or in the early morning and rarely induced by exertion. Women are more affected. and there is elevation of ST segment during the attack.

Unstable Angina : includes angina of recent origin angina, at rest or pre-infarction angina.

Treatment : The remedies will depend upon the expressions presented by the patient, it does not matter then what type of angina it is. General remedies which cover the pathogenesis of the Angina are: Amyl Nit., Arnica, Aurum met, Cactus, Spigelia, Latrodectus mactans, Lilium tigrinum.

Amyl nit.: the most striking symptom is deep facial flushing and pulsation all over the body with the palpitation of the heart. This is followed by drenching sweats. There is aching pain and constrictions around the heart with great anxiety. Precordial pain extends to the right arm. The pulse is strong and full.

Arnica: violent running, causing strain of the heart, palpitation and the pain extending to the left elbow and the arm. Heart pains travel from right to the left with stitching in the heart. There is constant fear of death with cardiac distress at night. The pulse is feeble and irregular.

Aurum met.: no other remedy produces more acute mental depression than Aurum met. Complaints after grief, fright, anger, disappointed love, contradiction, reserved displeasure, financial loss may bring on angina pains. There is sensation as if the heart has stopped beating. Heart feels bruised and sore, worse by suppressed foot sweat. The pulse is rapid, feeble, and irregular. Temporal and carotid arteries throb.

Cactus: is indicated where the heart is weak and arteries atheromatous. The chief action of Cactus centers around heart and circulation. It acts on the circular muscular fibers, hence there are constrictions. This is followed by general weakness and prostration. The constriction is as from the iron band. Palpitations are worse lying on the left side. At the approach of menses heart disease with the edema of the left hand. Usually useful in tobacco heart.

Spigelia: violent pains is the key-note of the remedial action. Violent palpitation that attend other symptoms. Throbbing of carotids and of subclavian arteries, violent sticking and compressive pains radiating to throat, arms, scapula, worse by least motion. Soreness, cracking and purring in the region of the heart. Whole left side is sore, pulse is intermittent and weak, stremulous, irregular. Better on lying on the right side.

Latrodectus mactans: affects the heart producing a typical picture of angina pectoris, restlessness with heart pains and prostration are the most important symptoms. Constriction of chest muscles radiating to the shoulders and back. This spider poison brings on a total degenerating effect on the blood. Precordial anxiety, and violent pains sharp and extending to shoulders or both arms to fingers with numbness. Feeble pulse that can be hardly counted.

Lilium tigrinum: has its main action on the venous circulation, the heart and the female organs. There is a sensation as if the heart is grasped in a vise. Feels clutched, full, bursting, cold, weak, hanging by thread. Palpitation, with the pain in cardiac region with a feeling of a load on chest, suffocation feeling in the crowded and in warm room. Pulse is rapid, irregular.

Management: In an acute attack, stop the exercise that the patient is undertaking. Put few drops Amyl nitrosum 3 on the tongue. There should be immediate relief. Reassure the patient that there is no immediate concern on his condition. Risk factors must be evaluated. Smoking should be stopped. Underlying condition like obesity, thyrotoxicosis and anaemia should be treated. Full history should be taken and regular treatment should be started.

4. ***Patient presents with history of sudden chest pain, similar in character to exertional angina pectoris, but has occurred at rest and which has remained for quite some time now. There is restlessness, occasional vomiting and sweating. The condition is MYOCARDIAL INFARCTION.***

Usually there are no abnormal physical signs unless any complications develop. There may be hypotension initially, and sinus tachycardia may develop. Diabetics, hypertensives and elderly patients have silent myocardial infarction. Myocardial infarctions may go unnoticed or may produce hypotension, breathlessness or arrhythmia.

Investigations to confirm the diagnosis of Myocardial infarction are necessary in order to determine the correct line of treatment.

Increased ESR and polymorpho nuclear leucocytosis may occur in the first few days following the MI attack. Necrotic cardiac tissues release cellular enzymes: Creatine kinase (CK), that peaks within 24 hours, and is back to normal in 48 hours.The size of the infarct determines the total enzyme release, and large infarcts tend to produce higher serum levels of enzyme. Serum glutamic oxaloacetic transaminase (SGOT), now known as Aspartate aminotransferase (AST) peaks at 24-48 hours and may fall within 72 hours to normal. AST is released by damaged red blood cells, kidney, liver and lungs. Lactic dehydrogenase peaks at 3-4 days and remains elevated till 10-14 days. Enzymes are usually estimated for first three days following a suspected attack. The first assay may be normal but the subsequent will be raised three to more fold rise. ECG is particularly important. The changes are seen in those leads where they face the infarct.

Treatment: Pain is the primary symptom that may need an immediate attention. Lethal arhythmia may occur. This needs special care and attention. Therefore it is always advisable to admit the patient to a coronary care unit of hospital as soon as possible. The emergency department must have the staff and facilities to provide the treatment required within the first few hours.

Before the patient is transported to the hospital one can prescribe **Morphinum** 3x-6x in frequent doses. It may take care of that restlessness, hyperesthesia, trembling, twitching and jerking of limbs; the patient becomes extremely susceptible to pain, which is the pathogenesis of this drug.

Arsenic alb: is another restless remedy that comes in the picture particularly when there is anxiety and constant fear of death. As the Infarct progresses, it may develop arrhythmia, either bradycardia or tachycardia. Ventricular extra systoles are common. Ventricular fibrillation may follow.

Digitalis: is a good heart remedy, where there is slow, irregular and intermittent pulse with dropsy of the internal and external parts. There is weakness and dilatation of the myocardium. The pulse is slow in recumbent posture but irregular and dicrotic in sitting posture. The greatest indication of Digitalis is when auricular fibrillation has set in and there is failure of compensation. There is coldness of skin, irregular respiration, bluish appearance of the face. There is sudden sensation of stoppage of heart (Opp Gelsimium). F, 3, 30 are commonly used.

Iberis amara: has dull or stitching pains, palpitation and breathlessness on slightest exertion. Pains radiate down the left arm and there is irregular pulse. Consciousness of the heart is the characteristic symptom. The pulse is full, irregular and intermittent. Slightest exertion, laugh, cough aggravates the situation. Wakes up in the morning at 2 a.m. with tachycardia. The concomitant symptom of heat and fullness in the head and neck, vertigo and nausea are very important. The excessive nervous and frightened condition with cold hands and feet frequently found associated with the heart condition is present.

Remedies mentioned under *Angina pectoris* can also be considered for Myocardial infarct. The death and the necrosis of the myocardial and coronary tissue is checked by these drugs and helps the heart to come back gradually to its normal working condition.

Oxygen at 60% is usually given routinely through face mask or nasal cannulae for several hours because during the acute attack of MI, the arterial PO2 is reduced.

Management

Bed rest is essential initially but, if possible, full mobilization should be achieved within a week or ten days to reduce the degree of physical and mental debility inflicted by this illness. Smoking should be stopped. 50% mobility can be allowed in a month's time depending on the rate of recovery. The patient can return to his normal work after 3 months. Car driving may be prohibited for 6 months.

5. ***A child or an young adult between the age of 5-15 years, suddenly comes with fever, fleeting joint pains, mostly the large joints like knee, elbow, ankles and wrist, that are swollen, red and tender; malaise and loss of appetite. The disease is probably ACUTE RHEUMATIC FEVER.***

Rheumatic fever is a disease that develops as result of infection with group A Streptococci. It affects the heart, skin, joints, and central nervous system. Pharyngeal infection with group A streptococcus may be followed by the clinical syndrome of Rheumatic fever. Clinically two major manifestations are seen : Cardiac features and non-cardiac features.

Cardiac features manifest as: New or changed heart murmurs, development of enlargement of the heart or a cardiac failure, development of pericardial effusion with ECG changes (raised ST segment) or myocarditis (inverted or flattened T-waves), a transient diastolic mitral murmur.

Non-cardiac features manifest as: fever with excessive tachycardia, a fleeting polyarthritis, Sydenham's chorea (spasmodic unintentional movements), Erythema marginata.

Investigations are necessary to come to a diagnosis. Throat swab culture for A Streptococcus. The anti-streptolysin O titre, Non-specific indicators such as ESR and C reactive protein levels (raised).

Treatment

Patient with fever, active arthritis or active carditis should be completely rested in bed. When the clinical syndrome has subsided (e.g. no pyrexia, normal pulse rate, normal ESR, normal leucocytic count) only then the patient may be mobilized.

Arsenic alb: is useful in a very early stage — the non-cardiac stage — prevails mostly with the fever, with excessive tachycardia, polyarthritic pains. It is invaluable in rheumatism, where the pains are shooting, burning and lancinating; great restlessness, peculiar thirst and extreme prostration.

If this phase is not recognized then the cardiac involvement may take place giving symptoms of burning, oppression about the heart with small, feeble and rapid pulse.

Apis mel: follows well especially when there is peculiar wax-like appearance of the swollen joint with prostration, fever, but without thirst, together with other concomitants.

Rhus tox: is valuable in every form of rheumatism. Its marked modalities point to the field of usefulness. There is pronounced weakness of limbs. Sense of stiffness on first moving the part after rest. Drawing and tearing pain in the limbs during rest. Shining swelling of the joints. Stitching pain in the heart with painful lameness and numbness of left arm. Arnica is one of the most valuable remedy in articular or muscular rheumatism arising out of traumatism or otherwise. Great prostration and sensitiveness to touch, sore bruised feeling is always present. Violent stitches in the left chest with pain in the inter-costal muscles.

Eupatorium perfoliatum: has great soreness of bones and muscles accompanied by perspiration. The pain is deep into the bones with sensation of broken bones. In whatever circumstances it may be present, aggravation is mostly in the morning and on moving.

Dulcamara: is very sensitive to cold and damp, this modality runs through this remedy. Changes from hot to cold induces rheumatic trouble. Great oppression of the chest, when breathing, dull shooting as if blows in and about the sides of the chest.

Rhamnus californica: has inflammatory rheumatism of joints, swollen and painful, has tendency to metastasis, has profuse sweat, and rheumatic heart.

"The word rheumatism conveys to the mind a general symptomatology of pain that is similar to certain characteristics whether the difficulty be gout, arthritis, inflammatory rheumatism, or any other disease syndrome, acute or chronic, or from whatever underlying cause, affecting certain group of tissues. The first principle of prescribing that the differentiation of the remedies lies not in the differences of the disease entities, but in the differentiation of modalities, and sensations and locations of parts or tissues affected." **H.A. Roborts.**

If the patient in non-cardiac features delays in presenting himself to the physician for treatment, the condition may transform to the cardiac state and present the picture as described earlier.

Adonis vernalis: acts predominantly on heart when it is affected after rheumatism, influenza or nephritis where the muscles of the heart are in a fatty degeneration : Wandering pains. It regulates the pulse and increases the power of contractions, with more urinary secretions. Useful in rheumatic endocarditis, mitral and aortic regurgitation and arrhythmia. Pre-cordial pain, palpitation, dyspnoea and marked venous engorgement. Also useful in myocarditis. There is not much literature on the use of this drug in potencies but it is mostly used in Mother tincture form.

Cactus grandiflora: chief action centers around the heart and circulation. There are constricting pains all over. Constriction as from an iron band, palpitation worse lying on the left side, endocarditis with mitral insufficiency, together with violent rapid action, murmurs, excessive impulse, increased precordial dullness, enlarged ventricles, low blood pressure, arteriosclerosis. Tobacco Heart.

Kalmia latifolia: affects the nerves, heart, circulation, a heart, nerve and rheumatic remedy. Heart's action is tumultuous, rapid and visible, paroxysm of anguish around the heart, fluttering of heart with anxiety, stabbing and sharp shooting pains, radiating to left scapula, palpitation worse while leaning forward. Frequent pulse. Tobacco Heart.

Lithium carb.: affects notably head, eyes, heart, small joints and urinary organs. Chronic Rheumatism connected with heart lesion, and uric acid diathesis. Trembling and fluttering in the heart, extending to back, throbbing and dull stitch in the cardiac region, pains in the heart before menses.

Spigelia anthelmintica: violent palpitations, audible throbbing of carotids, sticking and compressive pains radiating to throat. Rheumatic carditis, trembling pulse, whole left side is sore. Pulse is intermittent with palpitations weak tremulous irregular.

Whatever is the disease condition, Aconite is thought of only if there is typical restlessness, physical and mental, anxiety, and the complaints are caused by sudden exposure, suppression of sweat after influenza and colds: Stitching pains in the chest, palpitation with anxiety, shortness of breath, oppressed breathing. Cough is short and hacking — worse at night and after midnight. Pulse is fast, full, hard, tense and bounding.

Apis: has palpitation of the heart, heart stitches backward from the apex, and has scanty secretion of the urine. The pulse is hard, small, intermittent, and quick but weak. In fever, skin is dry hot, alternating with gushes of sweat. Thirstless. Useful when there is effusion.

Arsenic alb.: there is pre-cordial pain, that radiates to neck, and occiput. Pulse is more rapid in the morning, and there is palpitation with anguish. Difficult breathing, great fear of death, extreme restlessness, marked weakness, and lack of vital heat and night aggravation are the characteristics.

Bryonia: has typical affections of the serous membrane, dryness all over. Sharp stitching in the chest on coughing. The pulse is full and quick, modalities are important.

Kali carb: has violent palpitation, throbbing extends to the tip of the fingers, there is burning in the heart region, and the heart pains extend to the left scapula there is generalized weakness in the heart, limbs, back. Weakness of the intellect is also important. Suited to fleshy people, sensitive to atmospheric changes, to every draft of air, chilly and has a tubercular constitution.

Mercurius solubilis: is typical Hahnemann's anti-syphilitic remedy. Palpitation on slightest exertion, pulse is irregular, quick, strong and intermittent or soft or trembling.

Spigelia: is suited to more anaemic, debilitated, rheumatic and scrophulous subjects. Violent palpitations, audible, throbbing of carotids and subclavian arteries. Violent sticking and compressive pains, radiating to throat, arms, worse least motion. Pulse is intermittent with palpitation weak tremulous and irregular.

Spongia: has rapid and violent palpitation, with dyspnoea, awakened in the middle of the night with pain and suffocation, feels better in resting in horizontal position. There is right heart hypertrophy with asthmatic symptoms. Pulse is frequent, hard, full, or feeble. Sometimes symptoms of valvular insufficiency.

6. ***A middle-aged person with otherwise a normal disposition complains of irritability of mind on slightest provocation, weariness, tiredness or fatigue, mostly towards the evening. At times palpitation and dizziness is also present. Most probably he is suffering from HYPERTENSION.***

In majority of cases no cause can be identified, and this form of hypertension is called **Primary/Essential Hypertension.** Wherever the cause of hypertension can be established, that hypertension is termed as **Secondary Hypertension**. These cases are generally very small and about less than 10% cases.

There is no single factor that has been found to explain the Essential Hypertension. The increase in blood pressure is due to small increase in cardiac output. This is due to sympathetic over-activity. Later in the disease there is normal cardiac output but increase in peripheral resistance. Causes of this essential hypertension are numerous but the main ones are Genetic factor, Obesity, Intake of alcohol, Intake of excess of salt and smoking.

Secondary Hypertension should be considered more seriously in patients with blood pressure. Above 80% of patients of this variety are showing causes in the kidney and their function. This is probably because of salt and water retention. Endocrine causes. Includes Conn's Syndrome, Pheochromocytoma, Cushing's Syndrome, Acromegaly, Hyperparathyroidism, Cardiovascular causes, pregnancy pre-eclampsia, Diabetes mellitus and Drugs.

The primary rule to treat the hypertension is to identify the cause of the Hypertension in the individual and try to resolve the case.

Hahnemannian pathology classifies Hypertension into four classes in accordance with the Miasmatic break up:

Functional or Psoric Phase; Sycotic Phase; Tubercular or Pseudopsoric Phase; and Syphilitic or Destructive Phase.

In the Psoric or the functional phase the levels of blood pressure show constant fluctuation. It is, therefore, also known as Labile Hypertension. With passage of time and inadequate treatment this may pass into a regular hypertension. When regular appropriate treatment may be required. The main cause of this hypertension is Stress at both the emotional or physical level. Emotional disturbance such as Excitement, Anger, Anxiety, Worries, Tension, Shock due to financial loss, or loss of dear ones can seriously affect an individual which can result into rise in blood pressure. Pregnancy is a good example of physical stress that may raise the blood pressure. Physical overwork beyond one's capacity for a long period, inadequate rest and sleep can also tend to raise the blood pressure. But as soon as these stresses are over there is always a downward trend of blood pressure and they may attain a normal level. As long as no abnormal physical signs are demonstrable only change in attitude in life or change of life style is needed for normalcy. This can be brought about by counselling. To get angry, or to get anxious or tensed or develop worries or brooding etc., are inherent traits of the individual which have been built up over many years and even through the hereditary transmissions. We cannot get rid of them totally but we can certainly reduce their intensities through application of appropriate homoeopathic remedies and by counseling.

Treatment

Like any other case, a full case history and physical examination is essential to determine the cause of the elevated blood pressure. Often these cases are asymptomatic. Or may have mild headaches or occasional epistaxis and inadequate sleep or overwork with irregular eating habits. At times these patients are over-conscientious, or diligent or scrupulous. One needs a great perseverance to handle these persons.

Patient reveals in his history that he is going through some emotional disturbance, grief, or disappointment, has a mild headache towards the evening and cannot concentrate on his work and even has some sleepless nights and has become short- tempered and irritable. He has also turned introvert. Dwells constantly on the past unpleasant happenings. He wants to be alone and to cry but cannot. At this point wants no consolation. On examination shows tachycardia with elevation of blood pressure. One is reminded of Ignatia and Natrum Murriaticum. Emotional element interferes with the coordination of functions in Ignatia. Ailments from grief, fright or emotional shocks, disappointments, unhappy love, sighing and sobbing and inward weeping. Oversensitive and nervous and constantly frustrated. Worse from consolation. This hypersensitive emotional character causes headaches with throbbing and causes the congestive throbbing in the head in spots shifting from place to place, with increase in blood pressure. Anger and humiliation following a heated argument causes nervous disorders and irritability and trembling. Natrum mur is the chronic of Ignatia.

Staphysagria: very sensitive, morbidly sensitive, the least word that seems wrong hurts very much, special senses become irritable, cannot tolerate touch, odour, noise that sends the blood surging to the heart and head — causes the blood pressure rise. There is urinary complaint with the emotional state. Frequent desire to pass urine with burning in urethra. When not urinating, a feeling as if the bladder is not empty.

Belladonna: has one marked symptom of congestive headache, with throbbing, hot and red face with burning eyes. This may start after a head bath, or a hair cut that is relieved by tight bandaging. There is rise in systolic pressure with full bounding pulse. The blood pressure returns to normal after the congestion is normal.

Glonoin: has sudden and violent irregularities in circulation with sensations of pulsation throughout the body. Hyperaemia of the brain, congestive headaches, mostly due to suppressions of the menses, the shocks in the head are synchronous with the pulse. Better by elevating head and in open air. There is a characteristic mental condition "loss of sense of location". Like in Belladonna, exposure to sun, bright light, or working in heat or under gas-light, may also produce this hyperaemia. Slightest touch to the head or weight on the head causes headache.

We have seen the Psoric dimensions of the hypertensive expression caused because of the mental, emotional or physical stress.

These Psoric expressions get greatly exaggerated in Tubercular type of hypertension. These changes are highly fluctuating, and may even lead to epistaxis, bleeding from ears, eyes, nose etc. At times patient may present with these symptoms, in fact these symptoms often work as safety valves. Blood pressure measured at this point may show elevated figures. Immediate attention is therefore required.

Phosphorus: a tall person, slim and slender, of sanguine temperament, is ideally a tubercular personality. The bleeding here is due to fatty degeneration of tissue, and organs. Phosphorus is chilly and of tubercular diathesis. In tubercular personalities the symptoms are greatly accelerated and may produce cerebral oedema. Left ventricular failure or renal impairment. Retinal haemorrhages exudates and papilloedema, when present, are diagnostic of malignant hypertension, more and more complications are present and possible at this point.

Lachesis: another remedy that is important. Warm-blooded and highly susceptible personality, susceptible to emotions like grief, sorrow, fright, vexation, jealousy and disappointment in love. Being a hot patient always aggravated by hot weather, sun, hot drinks and warm rooms. Blood rushes to the head with throbbing pains leaving the extremities cold. Pulsation and hammering in the head, bleeding from any part of the body relieves the headache. Often found useful in menopausal complaints. Cardiac difficulty often associated with the headache.

Fagopyrum esculentum: is cross and depressed personality, and having inability to fix attention. There is throbbing in all the arteries with irregular pulse, palpitation and oppression. There is bursting headache.

The hypertension in Sycotic personality may be caused by the systemic disorders. The functional labile blood pressures, when unchecked, pass on to the changes in the body's biochemistry, resulting into changes in the diastolic pressure, either due to atherosclerotic changes in the blood vessels, or in the renal tissues. Metabolic changes in as Eonn's syndrome, Pheochromocytoma, Cushing's syndrome. Acromegaly or Hyperthyroidism or renal changes like chronic glomerulonephritis, chronic atrophic pyelonephritis, and congenital polycystic kidneys are the commonest causes. In fact, it is difficult to say whether the hypertension has caused the renal disease or vice versa. Hypertension in pregnancy in its early stages is the essential hypertension where-as in later phases it is pre-eclampsia which is accompanied by proteinuria and oedema. Inake of alcohol, certain drugs and smoking may cause hypertension. Appropriate treatment may have to be instituted depending on the systemic disorder that is present with the hypertension.

And finally, in the syphilitic dimension where there is organic damage has taken place, we are reminded of Aurum met.

Aurum met: it has increased force of circulation, with flushes of heat and followed by perspiration. Forceful beating of the heart, which may be irregular, easily quickened by noise, excitement or contradiction. Extra systoles are common, local pulsations are prominent. Desire for fresh air but covers the head when aching. It is usually a fatty heart, with hypertrophy associated with renal disease and cirrhosis of the liver in gouty subjects. Along with all this there is always a depressive mind. Because of disappointed love, contradictions, reserved pleasures, and financial losses.

Baryta mur: causes vascular degeneration causing hypertension with comparative high systolic pressure and low diastolic pressure. Present with cerebral and cardiac symptoms. There is accelerated heart beats with palpitation, and scarcely perceptible pulse that is irregular.

Management

Routine investigations of a hypertensive patient should include:

A chest X-ray; ECG; Urine analysis; Fasting blood sugar, Lipid profile; Urea and electrolytes.

A review of the patient's life-style and diet may suggest modifications of lifestyle that could lead to some reduction in blood pressure.

Weight reduction. Reduction in heavy alcohol consumption. Salt restriction. Regular exercise and meditation — these are the techniques that have shown reduction in blood pressure. An attempt should be made to reduce the stress and anxiety.

Patient should be educated in tying to treat themselves by observing the do's and don't's as suggested by the physician. It must be impressed on them that one single attempt at treatment does not cure hypertension. It is a long-drawn process of regular medication, regular check up and diet. Regular exercise, such as brisk walk for about 3-5 km per day, is equally essential as medical treatment.

7. ***A patient giving a history of rheumatic fever several decades earlier, recurrent bronchitis and progressively developing severe dyspnoea, productive blood-tinged sputum, and occasionally blood vomiting — frank haemoptysis — lower abdomen and limb swelling — the condition is MITRAL STENOSIS.***

There will be bilateral cyanotic or dusky pink discoloration over the upper cheeks, at first the pulse is regular but later there is irregular with atrial fibrillation. The apex beat is tapping in character, a diastolic thrill may be present. X-ray shows a small heart with enlarged left atrium. In sinus rhythm ECG shows bifid P wave. This double humped P is seen best in leads II, V3 and V4.

Laurocerasus: constriction of the chest, and burning in the chest on inspiration. Dyspnoea with sensation that he is unable to raise the chest walls, and is better lying down. Folds hand over the chest, as if there is some trouble there, worse by exercise. Pulse is weak and variable, slow or irregular. Clutching at heart and palpitation. Coldness is common sensation.

Strophantus: chronic nervous palpitation and arrest of breathing. Heart's action is weak rapid, irregular, due to muscular debility and insufficiency. Stitches and twitches at the apex. Mitral stenosis and regurgitation. The pulse is rapid alternating with slow, weak and irregular. Violent palpitations. Heart is greatly dilated, pulsation diffused, double mitral bruit, dullness at both the bases of the lungs. Moist rales, expectoration of bright blood, haemoptysis. Use in Mother tincture form.

Mild mitral stenosis may not need any treatment, other than prompt treatment for accompanying bronchitis. Mild dyspnoea can be treated with diuretics like Apocynum and Acetic acid. And if there is beginning of atrial fibrillation then use Digitalis. In case it continues to deteriorate surgical intervention is suggested.

8. ***Patient complains of fatigue and lethargy, a sense of palpitation, dyspnoea and develops arthopnoea. And on examination there is atrial fibrillation, having displaced systolic thrill, soft S_1 S_3 with pan-systolic murmur. The condition is MITRAL REGURGITATION.***

Crataegus oxycantha: acts on the heart muscles and is an excellent heart tonic. Useful in chronic heart disease with extreme weakness and oppression. Extreme dyspnoea on the slightest exertion. Incompetent vales with valvular murmurs. Pulse is accelerated, irregular, feeble, intermittent. Often there is cardiac dilatation. Arteriosclerosis is associated.

Strophanthus *(see above)*

Medorrhinum: it is a chronic sycotic and hydrogenoid drug. Used usually when there is chronic inflammation of the valve after the rheumatic fever. It is used normally as an intercurrent remedy.

Valvular diseases of the heart are congenital in nature or produced after the attack of rheumatism. Originally there is compensatory phenomenon and the treatment can help the patient when prescribed on the available signs and symptoms. But when the compensation fails then the treatment cannot do much to relieve the patient. As the compensation fails the signs and symptoms aggravate and go beyond the scope of medication. Surgical intervention is, therefore, necessary.

9. ***The patient complains of dyspnoea on slight exertion, and on examination the position of the apex beat is indefinite, the impulse is diffuse, the first sound is short and sharp, the condition is CARDIAC DILATATION.***

Here the systolic pump function of right or left ventricles is impaired. And these enlargements often produce symptoms of congestive cardiac failure. Dyspnoea on exertion is the primary symptom, fatigue, orthopnoea, paroxysmal nocturnal dyspnoea, and peripheral oedema, palpitations develop in due course. The prognosis of these patients is poor.

Crataegus oxycantha: acts on the muscles of the heart, and is an excellent heart tonic. It does not produce any cumulative action. Patient suddenly becomes weak, heart muscles seem flabby, worn out, oppression of the heart with weakness. Cardiac dyspnoea, and dropsy on slight exertion, without increase in the pulse. The pain is experienced under the clavicle .The heart is dilated with first sound weak. In order to achieve good results five to ten drops of the tincture should be employed over prolonged period.

Digitalis purpurea: Least movement causes violent palpitation. And sudden sensation as if the heart would stop. Irregular heart, specially if the mitral valve is involved. These cardiac conditions may start after fevers. Hypertrophy of the heart with dilatation. Pulse is weak and quickened by least movement. It is very slow at rest.

Phaseolus: Heart symptoms are quite pronounced. Irregular and weak pulse, breathing slow. The most important concomitant symptom is that the patient is diabetic. The palpitation is so vigorous that there is always a feeling that death is approaching. Curious feeling in the chest and at that time there is feeble and irregular pulse.

Cactus grandiflorus: It is a heart tonic, and this remedy benefits large number of weakened and painful hearts, and its keynote is constriction, with pain and numbness in left arm.

Phosphorus: is indicated when associated with the respiratory complications such as broncho-pneumonia, or pleuritis.

There may not be any cure to this enlargement but the distressing symptoms can be removed or reduced, and may stop further damage to the myocardium.

10. ***Apex beat is below its normal position, the impulse forcible and heaving, on auscultation, the first sound is dull and prolonged. This is the HYPERTROPHY OF HEART.***

Patient does not present any sign and symptom if the hypertrophy is well-compensated for the obstruction in the circulation, which has caused the hypertrophy; in fact he is unaware of any cardiac disorder. The enlargement is rarely in actual practice limited to one chamber of the heart. It is essentially a compensatory process. If the cause is removable then the prognosis is favourable. Actual physical examination of the patient can reveal the status of the heart.

Arnica montana: has fatty heart and hypertrophy, mostly due to excessive straining of the heart as in case of athletes — severe pain in the elbow of the left arm, distressing dyspnoea with cardiac distress, the heart muscles are weakened. On the basis of the same modality, Rhustox is also indicated. But has an odd symptom of coldness of the nose.

Aurum met.: the patient is hypertensive, with valvular lesions of arteriosclerosis. Develops a sensation of heart being stopped for couple of seconds, and restarts with tumultuous action. The pulse is rapid, irregular, and feeble.

Bromium has a similar cause as that of Arnica. Here there is hypertrophy due to gymnastics, violent palpitation, worse on lying on the left side. There is nervous palpitation with nausea with headache.

Kalmia lat: there is anguish around the heart, fluttering of the heart, with anxiety, palpitation is worse on leaning forward. The pulse is slow tremulous. Often we find these are smokers. They have also suffered from rheumatic fever. Worse from sunrise to sunset.

Lithium carb: It is considered in a case where there is history of chronic rheumatism, associated with the there is history of chronic rheumatism, associated with the cardiac lesions. Whole body feels sore and heavy. Two grand characters about the heart symptoms, worse on bending forward better after urinating, but worst on rising to urinate. Pain in the heart is usually before menses, at times.

11. ***Patient, usually an elderly, complains of severe cramping pain or discomfort in the legs while walking which disappears after a short rest, but recurs when the walk is resumed, the condition is INTERMITTENT CLAUDICATION.***

Intermittent claudication is caused by the peripheral arteriosclerosis including arterial thrombosis, this is often senile or diabetic. It is caused also by the inflammatory disease of the arteries like thromboangiitis obliterans or infection like subacute bacterial endocarditis, tuberculosis, syphilis, typhoid fever, or Polyarteritis nodosa, giant cell arteritis, rheumatoid disease etc. Intermittent claudication can also take place due to abnormal vasoconstriction — Raynaud's disease, or due to physical or chemical agents such as trauma, contusion, intravenous fistula or aneurysm; chilblain, frostbite, trench foot and immersion foot, Phenols, ergot etc.

The symptoms will be slightly varying depending on the site of obstruction, inflammation, or degeneration.

Treatment

With the typical symptoms of **Arsenic alb.** there is weariness and trembling of the limbs, and associated with the contraction of the limbs. Better by hot application, must move the limbs constantly or walk about. Restless feet.

Secale cornutum, has distorted limbs with paralytic condition, numbness and pricking sensation, paralysis develops after spasm, limbs are cold and there are cramps in the calves, gait is dragging. Icy coldness of the limbs. Skin is shrivelled, cold, wrinkled, dry or bluish development of slow dry gangrene. Wants parts uncovered.

Cactus grand. Has constrictive feeling, with acute pain. It is known for its use in aneurysm of large arteries and heart, weakness of the heart with arteriosclerosis. Alternate clutching and release feeling. Constricting pains run through the pathogenesis of this drug.

Management

Patient should be asked to refrain from smoking and if he has diabetes or hypertension he should control both the conditions. If obese, one should be asked to reduce weight. Limb must be kept warm but no local heat should be applied. Regular exercisers should be suggested for regularizing the circulation by development of anastomozing the vessels.

12. ***An elderly patient complains of painful, tender, cord-like structure, associated with redness and swelling, involving long saphenous veins often with varicosities. The condition is SUPERFICIAL THROMBOPHLEBITIS.***

Hamamellis: has principle action on veins of the rectum, genitals, limbs and throat producing venous congestion and haemorrhage. There is marked soreness of the parts, in fact it is bruised soreness and useful in post-operative care of pain. The haemorrhage is dark.

Vipera berus or (Syn. Vipera torva): in case of phlebitis and varicose veins is "worse on letting the affected limb hang down as if it would burst with fullness". There is inflammation of the veins with great swelling.

Fluoric acid: has characteristic destructive properties and, therefore, causes decay of long bones, ulcerations, bedsores and varicose veins. A remedy of old people with swollen scrotum and varicocele.

13 PREVENTION OF DISEASES AND PROPHYLAXIS

- Mission of the phyisician
- Role of the family physician
- Arndt's law
- Genus epidemicus
- List of Homoeopathic prophylactics

Physicians of utmost fame
Were called at once;
but when they came,
They answered as they took their fees,
'There is no cure for this disease'.

Hilare Belloc

Family doctor plays an important role in encouraging people to make full use of preventive services and in advising them about healthy living. But with industrialisation, population explosion, modernisation this institution of family doctor is gradually disappearing and instead more specialisation and specialist doctors are being turned out of medical institutions.

For patients of all ages it is the duty of the doctor to encourage healthy living habits, in matters such as exercise and diet with emphasis on energy value appropriate to the needs of an individual. This is possible only by the family physician who knows the ways, traditions, food habits of his patients with whom he is in constant touch.

In order to reach the scattered rural population a chain of health centres is needed. At these centres, health education is actively pursued along with maternity and child welfare.

Breast feeding of children for at least for the first six months should be advocated. Similarly, the importance in educating small children in methods of cleanliness and dental care should be insisted on.

The family doctor should carry on regular screening for diseases like tuberculosis, hypertension and diabetes mellitus. Healthy young women should be examined regularly for malignant diseases of breast and cervix, which can be detected at an early stage. Self-examination by women of the breasts can be taught and at the middle-age, women should be screened at regular intervals to facilitate early recognition of diseases. In fact the doctor should insist on more of preventive measures than curative in his practice.

From the very earliest period of the history of medicine until the most recent times, search for absolute preventives of diseases and for preservatives against poisoning has always occupied a large share of attention of those who occupied themselves with medical art (Dr. Dudgeon).

History informs us that varieties of preservatives have been announced in one age and despised and neglected in the next. Even at present we see that the Roman Catholic Church arrogates for itself a monopoly in the manufacture of amulets and charms in the shape of crucifixes, images of saints, medals and rosaries. We in India also subscribe to the same thought process by wearing red thread around the wrist, using chains with pendants of the images of their deity, saints and or prophets.

In recent times attempts have been made — with more or less success — to discover prophylactics. One of the most noted and successful of these is the introduction of vaccination by Jenner, in 1798, as prophylactic of small pox which worked to a marvellous extent. In fact it has almost wiped out small pox from the face of the earth. Recent drive to immunize children below 5 years of age through Oral polio vaccine (OPV) has attracted our attention. We have almost eliminated polio from India. There are also vaccines like DPT, MMR, which are given to newborn and growing children according to preplanned schedules.

Improvement in the methods of hygiene has created an awareness in the mind of the public at large and medical men in particular. Hygienic prophylactics have greatly helped to reduce the incidence of diseases.

Rule that guides a homoeopathist to the selection of remedy should also lead him to the discovery of prophylactic. The *priori* discovery of such prophylactic is scarcely possible for the members of the modern medical personnel.

The first and the most celebrated of the prophylactics discovered by Hahnemann was the prevention of scarlet fever in its early stages.

Hahnemann's another observation was the use of Cuprum 30 taken once a week during the prevalence of the epidemic of cholera.

Dr. Hering, in 1830, suggested that the prevention of many diseases might be found in their own morbid products.

Dr. Croserio proposes a prophylactic against infection with gonorrhoea — Mercuris 30, three globules, taken on three successive nights after the suspicious contact, because of the analogy of the pathogenetic effect of gonorrhoea.

Dr. Winter, in his very learned eassy on prophylaxis, says that those chiefly liable to epidemic, miasmatic and contagious diseases are such as are not in a good relative state of health, there is something wrong in their vegetative system, to which these diseases have peculiar affinity. He adds that if this defective system is corrected and eradicate the faults we can put these persons in a condition to resist these diseases.

In order to effect these changes he proposes to give succesive doses of the 1st, 2nd and 3rd dilution or trituration of mercurius, followed by Sulphur, Calcarea, Lycopodium, Graphites, Aresenic.

If the mother is unhealthy during the gestation of the child we should devote great attention to her treatment, as by rendering her healthier, this will greatly influence the good constitution of their foetus. Hahnemann has suggested to give Sulphur in potency to the mother in order to free the foetus from Psora — the king of diseases.

"Prevention is better than cure". Homoeopathy is the science of therapeutics and works on the law of Similars. In other words, the cure takes place on the principle of "Let Likes be treated by Likes".

For treating patients through Homoeopathy the primary requirement is the availability of signs and symptoms as observed by the physician and as gathered from the patient after close questioning, respectively. In the absence of any sign and symptoms it is difficult to arrive at any remedy.

"Drugs selected as remedies on the homoeopathic principle act by stimulating the reserve antidotal powers of the body as does a vaccine. The tissues acted upon are those involved in the disease process of the case in hand, or those adjacent or analogous to them." (Neatby and Stonham).

Vaccines are used to stimulate the body mechanism even when the active disease is not present and in this manner is produced an abundance or superabundance of specific antibodies – a state of immunity against a particular disease being thus established.

In the same manner it is believed that there are few instances of the drugs exerting a similar prophylactic effect. For example, Belladonna against Scarlet fever, Thuja and Tartar emetic against small pox. We have also seen the effect of Arnica and Phosphorus before an operation to lessen shock and chloroform sickness, respectively. In order to increase sufficient stimulation and to reduce the tissue resistance, small doses must be used.

Arndt's law which is emphasized by Professor Schulz of Greifswald University and is expressed by Wheeler in following terms: ***"Small stimuli encourage life activity, medium to strong stimuli tend to impede it; and very strong stimuli to stop or destroy it."*** It explains that the drugs in different doses act differently. But they act differently in health and disease owing to the altered sensitiveness to stimuli in the case of diseased tissue.

Large number of cases are required to prove the preventive power of any agent. Although examples are provided in the case of cowpox, vaccination against small pox, and inoculation of vaccines in case of typhoid, both these are homoeopathic procedures — drug prophylaxis has not been tested under condition which suffice as proofs to a searching mind. Organized research in this matter is beyond the resources of our investigators. It is the government that deals with the method of prevention of disease and those who are involved in its planning and execution are required to be convinced of this approach.

Allen Sutherland mentions the efficacy of the homoeopathic prophylactic remedies for various conditions has not been proved by controlled studies and statistical records yet generation of homoeopaths have used these remedies in these conditions and they claim to have done it successfully. Their efficacy can be accepted even when they are not proved.

Stearns says "There is no doubt about the antibody formation induced by drugs. The drug that most closely stimulates the disease in all its clinical aspect is more likely to be a prophylactic than one less similar. "In case of epidemics the best prophylactic will be the remedy "Genus epidemicus" obtained by examining typical symptoms from the accurate observations of the first few cases. For all other conditions sought to be prevented, any remedy known to produce the identical condition suffices.

Regarding the potency to be used for such a procedure there is a wide variation of thoughts and opinions. Grimmer considers that very high dose of the 10M affords protection throughout the epidemic. Wheeler and Kenyon write that a dose of 30th potency of the prophylactic remedy will protect at least for a fortnight.

In our daily practice, we see many diseases in epidemic or endemic state, many conditions which need to be prevented in future either in the same patient or in the community that one stays in.

Measles and Chicken pox are one of the commonest of eruptive fevers that affect the children. Public health authorities have introduced plans of immunizing these children through immunization schedules. Similar immunization schedules are also planned for Diphtheria-Pertussis, Tetanus, Tuberculosis, Hepatitis, Parotitis, Poliomyelitis.

Homoeopathic prophylaxis

MEASLES	Bryonia, Aconite, Arsenic Pulsatilla.	Boericke
	Morbillinum 1M	Schmidt, Allen
	Pulsatilla	Ruddock
GERMAN MEASLES	Pulsatilla	
CHICKEN POX	Ant. Crud, Pulsatilla, Rhustox	Mackenzie
DIPHTHERIA	Apis 30;	Denman, Boericke.
	Diphtherinum 10M	Schmidt, Allen, Tyler
	Laccaninum,	Tyler)
	Merc cynatum	Fergie Woods, Grimmer
WHOOPING COUGH	Allium sativa, Pulsatilla	Lehman
	Coqueluchin	Clarke
	Drosera	Boericke, Grimmer
	Carbo veg, Cup met, Drosera	
	Pertussin	Grimmer
TETANUS	Ledum, Thuja, Arnica, 10M	Schmidt, Hendrson
		Patrick
	Hypericum	Boericke

TUBERCULOSIS	(Inherited) Tuberculinum bovinum	Burnett
	10M-50M-CM Two doses at long	
	intervals of each	Kent
HEPATITIS	Carduus mar.	Burnette, Proell
	Chelidonium	Galen, Dioscorides
	Myrica	Thomson
PAROTIDITIS	Partidinum	Allen, Schmidt
		Trifolium repens Boericke
POLIOMYELITIS	Lathyrus Sativa	Grimmer
	Bell, Gel, physostigma	Tyler, Smith
INFLUENZA	Influenzinum hispanicum 200	Schmidt
	Gelsemium	Fergi woods

Apart from these conditions, we see many circumstances where we need to employ prophylactic remedies. Such as:

SEA SICKNESS	Cocculus ind. 6x/12 three times a day prior to the journey.	
	This is useful for car sickness or motion sickness too.	
	Petroleum 6x is also found useful.	
AIR HUNGER IN THE HILLS	Coca 30	Farington
RADIUM BURNS	Phos	Grimmer
	Cadmium iodide	
SURGICAL SHOCK	Prior to the operation or Tooth extraction:	
	Arnica mont 30/200	Foubister
	Just a day earlier and prior to the operation.	
	Calendula Lotion 20 drops in pint of water	
	Externally : Staphysagria, specially before tooth extraction.	
X-RAY BURNS/ ILL EFFECTS	Acid Flour, Phosphorus, Silicea	Grimmer
	Cadmium iod.	
FEAR OF EXAMINATION	Argentum nit, Gelsemium	Henderson
	Patrick	
ALCOHOL CRAVING	Quercus, Sterculia, Sulphuric acid	Boericke
SMOKING TOBACCO	Tabacum, (high), Caladium	Grimmer
	Acid Nicotinic	Morgan
TOBACCO CRAVING	Caladium	Boericke
CALCULI FORMATION	Fragaria	Boericke
	China	Clarke
	Carduus mar	Karo
CALCULI FORMATION IN BLADDER	Hydregia, Lyco	Pierce
OPIUM ADDICTION	Berberis vul	Boericke

We are in the 21st century and the science has advanced so much that many methods to ascertain the immunities and development of antibodies are available. In fact, Homoeopathy should be able to answer many problems through these methods and techniques. These will help to resolve many unsolved questions.

With the creation of separate department for ISM under the Ministry of Health this should be possible.

Bibliography

Allen, Henry *J Chronic Miasms*

Clarke, J N *Dictionary of Practical Materia Medica*

Close, Stuart *The Genius of Homoeopathy*

Dudgeon, R E *Lectures on the Theory and Practice of Homoepathy*

Farrington *Comparative Materia Medica*

Hahnemann, Samual *Organon of Medicine*

Hampel, Charles J *Bachr's the Science of Therapeutics*

Hughes, Richard *Priciples and practice of Homoeopathy*

Murphy, Robin *Homoeopathic Medical Repertory*

Homoeopathic Remedy Guide

Neatby, Stonham *Manual of Homoeo Therapeutics*

Raue, G C *Special Pathology and Digionostic Therapeutics*

Sankaran, P *Prophylactics in Homoeopathy*

Some exciting gifts are up for grabs with this book!!

Textbook of Homoeopathic Therapeutics

With Clinical Approach

Dr K. P. Muzumdar

FREE Gifts Rs. 1000/-

Dear Readers

By now you must have gone through this book in the entirety. So we invite your assessment on this title with absolute impartiality and candid observations. After all, we publishers blindly depend on your benchmarking. Friends, please fill up the open spaces below with CAPITAL LETTERS. You may add some extra sheets of paper if the space provided is not sufficient for you.

i. What are the important topics of your syllabus which are not adequately covered in this book?

ii. In which chapters and on what topics the treatment of the subject-matter by the author is not satisfactory and why?

iii. Have you come across the typos, factual inaccuracies, inconsistencies, and other forms of mistakes in the book? If yes, then please specify the mistakes and page numbers.

iv. Name top three books on the same subject, which, in your consideration, are better than this book. Could you provide some reasons?

Your 1st Preference: ....

Your 2nd Preference: ....

Your 3rd Preference: ....

v. Any suggestion to improve the quality of illustrations, diagrams etc.?

vi. How did you like the cover design? Any suggestions on colours?

vii. Suggestions for further improvement of production standard:

viii. Who recommended you this book:

☐ Teacher ☐ Friend ☐ Parents ☐ Bookseller ☐ Librarian

ix. Name of the person who has recommended:

Designation: ....

Address: ....

Phone No.: ....

e-mail: ....

x. Name and address of the bookseller from whom you have purchased this book:

....

....

....

xi. Name and address of the library where you would like to find the book:

....

....

xii. Name and address of your institution (Please mention the University or Board):

....

....

xiii. Your name, e-mail, and complete postal address:

....

....

....

xiv. A few other titles published by us that you would like to read:

....

....

The best assessment will be rewarded half-yearly. The award will be in the form of our publications, as decided by the Editorial and Marketing Operations Division, amounting to Rs. 1000/- (Rupees one thousand) only.

....

Please mail the filled up coupon at your earliest to :

Editorial & Marketing Operations Division

NEW CENTRAL BOOK AGENCY (P) Ltd

8/1 Chintamoni Das Lane, Kolkata 700 009

West Bengal, INDIA

Ph. No.: 033 + 22418411, 22418573, 22419094

Fax: 033 + 22419573, 22413852

e-mail: ncbapvtltd@eth.net, ncba@cal2.vsnl.net.in

Website: www.centralgroup.com